The Broth of Oblivion
A True Story of a Mother and her Dementia

By Brian Morgan

Other books by Brian Morgan

The Richest Man in Persia
Wealth, Success <u>and</u> Happiness

You are Already Rich
Or How to be Rich Without Money

The Life of Jude
Saint of the Impossible

The Saint of the Impossible
Everything you wanted to know about St Jude

The True Christmas Spirit
Let Peace and Joy Fill your Heart
(Incorporating *The Legend of the Christmas Prayer*)

The Legend of the Magi Scrolls
Timeless Christmas Classics

All books available at amazon.com.
Details at brianmorganbooks.com.

The Broth of Oblivion

A True Story of a Mother
and her Dementia

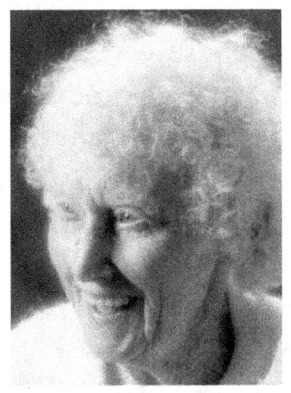

Brian Morgan

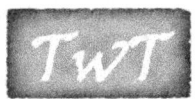

This book is associated with the website www.brianmorganbooks.com. A new Kindle eBook version of this book is available, as are eBooks in other formats (see the website).

This edition is presented in Australian English.

Printed under the CreateSpace imprint for the publisher and available online through amazon.com.
ISBN-13: 978-1511404860
ISBN-10: 1511404868

*In legend, the Broth of Oblivion
causes a soul to forget or to confuse
the details of its previous existence,
and eliminates memory of language,
so that words become a jumble.
The broth does not rid the soul
of its human feelings, however,
and it must suffer for previous sins
by knowing the degradation
of its present state.*

Contents

All sorrows can be borne
if you put them into a story
or tell a story about them.
Isak Dinesen.

Dedication

To the memory of
Kathleen Patricia Morgan,
my mother,
whose memory failed progressively,
especially in her later years,
until, finally, her heart failed
on All Saints' Day,
1st November, 2002.
Those who knew her might say
that this was a most
appropriate date.

To mum,
who represents the many lost souls like her.
And to those loving souls,
like my wife, Judy,
who care for them.

Author's Note

THE thoughts in this book ought to be private, and not for general consumption. They are about my mother and her dementia (Alzheimer's disease) and my memories of the last two years of her life.

However, when I wrote a short piece for her memorial booklet, people asked if I would develop the piece and perhaps have it published - not so much for those with dementia, who may not be able to focus on it, but for their families and carers (care-givers).

Carers need to know that they are not alone, and that they are not to blame for how the patient acts or feels. They need to know that guilt and depression are part of the journey, but that so are love and caring. They need to know that the guilt and the depression will pass, but the love will not.

This is what I must, and do, believe.

I used to play a little game with mum - and I think she saw it as a game - in which I looked for, and pointed out, something of beauty. It turned her thoughts from herself and brought a smile to her face.

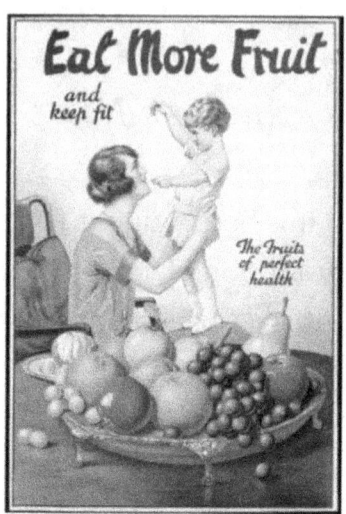

To care for those
who once cared for
us is one of the
highest honours.

*Tia Walker, The
Inspired Caregiver*

If these words can turn the thoughts of those involved with dementia (or simply old age) away from the shadows, it will be worth the pain of exposing private thoughts. If some of these words can induce a smile, so much the better. But even shedding a tear can help those whose heart is breaking, so I will hide nothing of importance. Above all, I hope I can help bridge the gap of understanding.

I am a journalist and author, but this is by no means an objective, journalistic view of dementia. Nor is it a clinical observation. It's just a personal perspective that might shed some light. I know I suffered, as millions are suffering, as, perhaps, you are suffering, and I came out the other end - as can you.

Although it took me quite a while to bring myself to write and eventually publish this, it seemed to me that, if I let the pen talk, and not the head, something might result that just might ease the suffering of others.

Enough of why I wrote. The book should speak for itself. It is written, in part, in short bursts, as a person with dementia thinks, and as those who care for them begin to think.

Forgive me if I've concentrated on my part in all this. I felt it had to be very personal. I haven't spoken much of my father, who passed away at 92, four years after mum. Mum made it to within three weeks of their 65th wedding anniversary. Mum was everything to dad. I can't speak of what her illness did to him - I think you would know. And he had suffered a stroke just a month before mum's collapse into her final illness. He was never the same after she went.

We could not care for mum at home for very long. She had to be in a secure nursing home because she was a "wandering" dementia sufferer. For her own safety, she had to be behind locked doors, despite our guilt and our shame. Mum and dad had moved to live with my wife, Judy, and me in their final years, but mum managed only a few months with us.

He was a tough man, my dad, and he kept his feelings to himself. I have respected this, but, as it turned out, I've had no choice in the matter. I was not able to consult with him during this writing, although I was his legal guardian. In January 2003, he was abducted from Camden Hospital, south of Sydney.

After police enquiries, the abductors turned out to be other family members, who took him nearly eight hundred miles away to north of Brisbane. God knows how he survived the journey in his state of health, but

I was unable to bring him back for the same reason he should not have gone - his health would not allow it.

So I lost a mother *and* a father. And I've lost other family members, some of whom may have tasted the broth of oblivion.

Putting all of that aside, I would need a bigger book than this to speak of Judy's role in mum's final two years. It was Judy who kept all communication lines open - to relatives, friends, and the three hospitals and two nursing homes involved. It was Judy who was best able to distract mum when she turned to anger or tears. It was Judy who was there for almost every visit, brushed mum's hair, trimmed and cleaned her nails, labeled her clothing, rubbed cream into her skin, treated her sores, washed her soiled clothes - did everything one heart can do for another.

It was Judy who kept dad and me going - we were in poor health ourselves. It is Judy who keeps me going still. And this from a woman who was treated shamefully by both mum and dad for many, many years. They, and my siblings, could never accept her as part of the family - and Judy and I have been married for a long time (6th April 1963).

Without Judy, those two years of caring for mum

and dad would have been impossible to contemplate. Her part in caring for both of them was much greater than mine, despite what it did to her own health (she suffered heart and immune system problems of her own in the end), and my love for her is beyond words.

For this book, I have tried, on occasion, to get into mum's head - and her thoughts are in italics.

If you are a carer, or care-giver, I wish you strength, persistence, and love. At the end of every long night, there *is* a dawn.

Gifts for the Treasure House

HOW extraordinary are the gifts of memory? And, as with so many beautiful things in mum's life, how she took them for granted. And don't we all?

So bountiful are these gifts of memory that mum rarely gave them a thought. Like the shepherd who sees ten thousand sunrises, but hardly notices one, she rarely paused to count her considerable blessings. She tended more to count the blessings of others. Pity.

The only time she gave memory much thought was when it failed her - and then she railed at it because she wanted it to be perfect.

"How silly I am," she thought aloud once. "Lord knows, a perfect memory would not be a blessing, would it? Perhaps it would be a curse."

So she knew, deep down, that a perfect memory was the last thing she would want, or the Good Lord would want for her. Some things are best forgotten.

You have to begin to lose your memory, if only in bits and pieces, to realize that memory is what makes our lives. Life without memory is no life at all, just as an intelligence without the possibility of expression is not really an intelligence. Our memory is our coherence, our reason, our feeling, even our action. Without it, we are nothing.

Luis Bunuel

She always hungered after material riches, but never attained them. Did she ever, even remotely, consider that the greatest treasure house in the world was the heart that beat within her? And that the thing that filled this treasure house and made it so rich was... memory?

I once gave her a manuscript I had written about this and many other things, hoping that she might give more credence to the written word than to the spoken.

The doctor, I wrote, sees the heart as a small muscle that pumps precious blood through our bodies to keep us alive. As long as it beats, we will live. The poet, on the other hand, sees the heart as a miracle of infinite size that pumps out precious love to keep other hearts alive. As long as it beats, our loved ones will live, if only in our memory.

Both doctor and poet are right, I wrote. The heart feeds on blood to preserve life, but it also feeds on memories to create love.

Ah, the memories mum stored in this infinite treasure house. The beauty of many sunsets, the smell of overdone onions, the sound of a wing flutter, the cluck of hens in a chook-house, the taste of ripe mango, the touch of her baby's skin, the heartbeats of a

If any one faculty of our nature may be called more wonderful than the rest, I do think it is memory. There seems something more speakingly incomprehensible in the powers, the failures, the inequalities of memory, than in any other of our intelligences. The memory is sometimes so retentive, so serviceable, so obedient; at others, so bewildered and so weak; and at others again, so tyrannic, so beyond control! We are, to be sure, a miracle in every way; but our powers of recollecting and of forgetting do seem peculiarly past finding out.

Jane Austen, Mansfield Park

lifetime. All stored in the treasure house.

If she had only thought about it, she would have realized that anything man or God can create can be stored as memories.

Anything. Good or bad.

She could have stored, and probably did store - despite her efforts to ignore them - grief and hurt, sadness, fear, hatred, guilt, bitterness, and all kinds of memories that bring pain to the heart and make it shrivel. Lord knows, I probably did enough, over the years, to cause her plenty of grief.

But, if she had embraced such feelings more, perhaps she would not have seen them as totally bad. Is not grief a measure of love, hurt a measure of health, sadness a measure of joy?

And does not memory - imperfect, but miraculous memory - take the edge off things negative and ease the pain, just as it can enhance joy or make the positive as perfect as we want it to be?

If she *had* thought about memory when she was able, she would surely have realized that it can distort, manipulate, blend, soften, harden, hide, and make the not-so-beautiful past beautiful. Surely she would have thanked God that memory is not absolutely perfect.

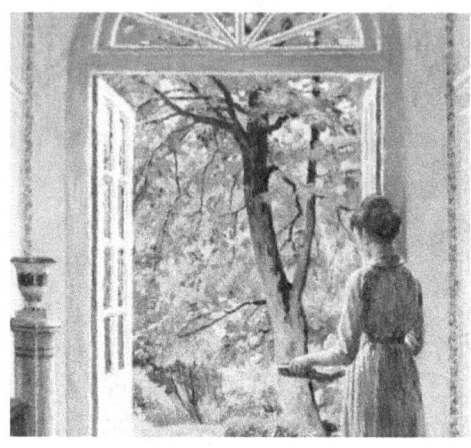

But the great paradox of memory is that it can bring tears of sadness or of happiness to the eye. It can help us relive past failure or past success. It can save us from mistakes and make us soar as we recall exhilaration and joyous times. It can pull all the strings of our emotions and activate all our senses.

For mum, though, it was very, very selective - as I guess it is for many of us. We all forget things that don't matter to us, but we also, by chance and by design, forget things that really do matter. Without even thinking about it, mum could push unpleasant memories to the backroom of the treasure house, and keep the beautiful thoughts in the living room. And she did so, deliberately and consciously, all her life - enough to preserve her well-being.

She would shudder and shake herself, as if forcing unpleasant thoughts to go away and be replaced by those more comfortable, more peaceful.

Thus, she selected and enhanced beautiful memories, rather than ugly ones, building wealth in the treasure house and love in the heart.

And, really, who can blame a gentle soul for accepting the positive and rejecting the negative? For looking to the light, rather than the shadow? For looking for the good, rather than the bad?

If you had suffered, as she had suffered, hardship of many kinds, if you had started a family in the uncertainty and horror of war, if you had seen your husband badly injured in an explosion and seen your brother come home from war without his face, and seen him die, as she did, and battled soul-crushing poverty, and nursed your mother through the wretchedness of dementia - if you had lived through such times, would you not also try to put up defenses?

Could you blame her for taking to her heart whatever serenity she could find in a harsh world? Or for letting beauty of thought be her guide in life?

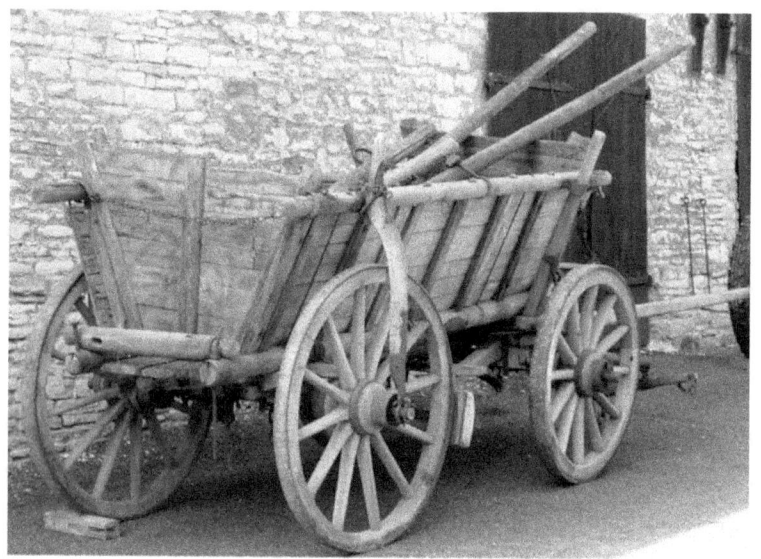

The days of horse and cart delivery.

Spring, Summer, Autumn...

THE spring of a girl's life should be a gondola ride of happiness, and, although life has a way of roughing the waters, mum and her family conspired to make the ride, if not entirely happy, then at least tranquil.

Mum came bellowing into the world in 1914, when the first guns were roaring in the War To End All Wars. But, with doting parents, plus four older sisters and two brothers, she would always be shielded in her childhood from anything remotely nasty.

In the days of horse and cart delivery of ice, milk, bread, rabbits and clothes props, life in the rambling, unpainted, weatherboard house in Sydney was difficult because of poverty, but serene because they all made it so.

"Rabbit-O," the vendor would yell as his horse clopped down the street, and all was right with the world.

A true friend can see the words in your heart and tell the story of your life when your memory is gone.

Tamara Artemis

God was good and the source of all blessings, especially to a red-headed, freckle-faced girl who went to a school and a church named after a saint called Mel. Some kids called it St Smell's, but little Kathleen never would, for fear of going straight to hell. The nuns were absolutely clear on that point.

It was in St Mel's school that mum first battled the demons of arithmetic - a battle she would relive many times in her years of confusion. For little did anyone realize at that time, mum's mother, my grandmother, had drunk of the Broth of Oblivion and had given it to several of her children, including her youngest, to sip.

The word "dementia" was virtually unknown in those endless days of blue skies and placid souls. Those were the days of picnics and parties and boating on a river you could walk on now, so thick is the pollution. Times have changed.

Mum met her "beau" on a tennis court on a joyous day of hit-and-giggle, and her backhand was so funny, he still chuckled over it nearly seventy years later. But he knew, straight away, "she was the one", and, after subjecting him to the ultimate test, a good sniffing by Boska, a pup of unknown, but suspect lineage, mum allowed herself to be smitten.

There is an old sepia photograph of the courting couple taken one week after they met. They had taken the ferry ride across Sydney Harbour to Manly Beach and were strolling on the promenade. Norman, my dad, the boiler-maker and champion footballer, was decked out in his Sunday best - three-piece suit, fob-watch dangling, hat, shoes you could see your face in, handkerchief tucked, just so, into his breast pocket. Mum, the stenographer and later gourmet food manager of a prestigious retail store, flowed in an ankle-length frock of frills and lace, gloves, hat, handbag, stockings - a picture of elegance and femininity. No-one would have known it, but, for each, it was their one and only set of good clothes.

The picture told the story. Already dad had slotted, with ease and a feeling of belonging, into the comfortable world mum had created - a world of beauty, harmony, gentility.

This was springtime, and no cloud dared creep over the horizon.

#

AFTER two years of frugal, but respectable courtship,

they were wed, on Boxing Day, 1937, in as grand a style as mum's father could afford. In a sign of how they were to live their lives, they chose not to have a honeymoon, but to use the money as a deposit on a house. Thus, they spent their wedding night under their own roof - and under a grand plan to control the summer of their lives, as mum had controlled her spring.

But early summer brings its storms.

In a far-off land, storm clouds gathered with frightening speed and rolled over land and sea until all but primitive societies were caught in the gloomy shadows of what people called the Great Depression.

Mum lost control and they lost their house. They were stunned. It was the first maelstrom of their life together and it was savage, unrelenting. But they proved resourceful and resilient and they weathered the storm - as they would weather many others in the years to come. As this and other storms passed, mum and dad never mentioned them again. These things were in the past, and unpleasant, and best forgotten.

In 1940, as the guns of World War II tore Europe apart, I arrived on the scene, their first-born. It was, I am told, a prolonged birthing that should have destroyed any urge for more children, but it did not. Three more children were to round out the family.

While mum was bringing life into the world, her thoughts must have turned to her brother, Bert, who, on the other side of the world, had played his part in destroying life in the first World War. But the unspeakable horrors of wartime were never mentioned on the beautifully embroidered postcards that traced Bert's passage through World War I.

Especially in times such as these, he had wanted to protect his much younger sister. However, an indiscriminate hand grenade knew nothing of his efforts to shield her, and blew half his face away. He came home, but died soon after, leaving a scar on mum's heart she could never truly forget, though a new World War made her try so very hard.

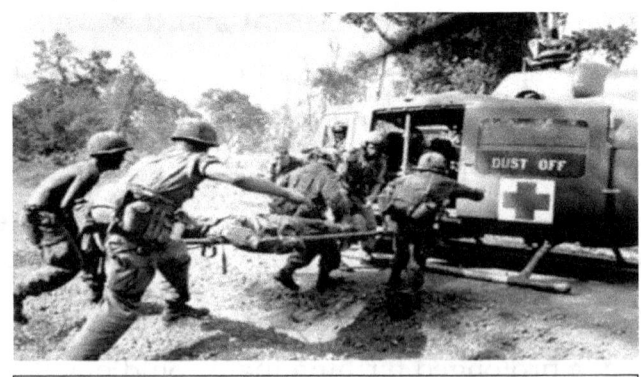

The unspeakable horrors of wartime.

She tried to never mention his name again, but, years later, when the Broth of Oblivion had fully poisoned her mind, she thought of Bert often - confusing him with me. Perhaps Bert's death opened up a tiny crack in mum's mind, letting the Broth of Oblivion seep in, because, after that, the tell-tale symptoms of dementia began to surface.

Pity the poor headmaster who called her in to complain about my misdemeanors. She never questioned me, though I was usually guilty as sin. She mercilessly brow-beat the bewildered headmaster, assuming the poor man had made another blunder. Obviously, *her* son could do no wrong.

The same fate befell a neighbor who had grabbed me after I had, allegedly, tried to blow up his letterbox with a fire cracker. Somehow the Broth of Oblivion made it all the neighbor's fault.

Aprons became mum's specialty. She would sew and embroider them to the absolute n^{th} degree of perfection for school fetes, never failing to soak up the gushing accolades she craved. She made toffees and toffee apples for the same fetes, throwing out batch after batch that had not attained perfection.

Much, much later, the family came to understand

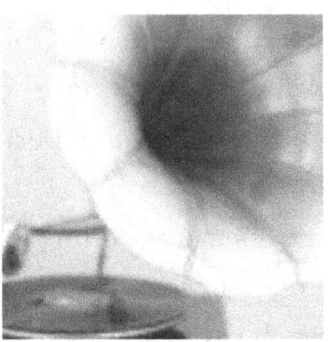

My memories pale as I prevail upon them again and again. They become more and more ghostly. I fear nothing so much as losing them altogether and having only my blank endless mind to live in.

E. L. Doctorow

that the striving after perfection and glory can be early signs of dementia. There was always the lounge room, for example, unsullied by children's feet - a room used *only* for visitors, so that they could leave with the vision of a perfect household. I believe, to this day, that only the Queen and the Pope were worthy of this room - and neither saw fit to visit.

And, where there was no perfection and no glory, mum tried to create it, lying about the achievements of husband and children, stretching the truth, exaggerating the reality. She always thought she was absolutely right to do such things, because, if things were not exactly as she said they were, then, of course, they should be.

Names were an increasing nightmare. Time after time, she would run through the long list of family names until, finally, annoyed and frustrated, she hit on the one she wanted. Next came the mixing up of names - calling someone by the wrong name and not realizing it. Then came the forgetting of names until gently reminded, and, finally, the remembering of names only from the distant past.

Short-term memory loss became a reality of life. Mum couldn't remember things that had happened minutes before. She'd ask the same question over and over. She'd forget what was on the stove, or that the stove was on.

Yet, in other ways her memory was "perfect", even if what she was "remembering" had never happened. I came across a quote from François, Duc de la Rochefoucauld (1613-1680): "Why can we remember the tiniest detail that has happened to us, and not remember how many times we have told it to the same person?"

In her mind, mum would create a story, perhaps combining elements of different stories into one and making something up to fill the gaps or to create the perfect story. Then she would tell this long, long story in minute detail, becoming angry and frustrated if she was interrupted. She would forget her place in the story, and, even if reminded, she'd start again from the beginning - not a word, not an inflection out of place.

And she would tell the same story, over and over, even if she was reminded of the previous telling. Out would come the whole story again, word for word, and the hapless audience would have to pretend they'd never heard that fascinating, perfect story before.

The Aboriginal people in Australia have a way of

escaping from the hardship of life and of forgetting their troubles. They "go walkabout". They simply take off, walking through the bush or the outback or along the ancestral songlines until the heart and the head are clear and they are ready to come back.

Some people with dementia, including mum, also go walkabout. With them, it's less a conscious decision to escape or forget, but simply a forgetting. They forget where they are and where they are going. They forget time. They just forget.

Thus mum would go walkabout. She'd slip away from church or shopping and charge off in the wrong direction. Family members would have to watch her all the time, because she was so swift of foot.

Sometimes it was not just a matter of going walkabout, of forgetting. Sometimes, when the stress of seeking tranquility and perfection in an imperfect world became too great, she would take off, almost at a run, and, if no-one saw her go, it would become a police matter to find her, with family members scattering in all directions to help in the search.

Dementia sufferers who go walkabout are called "wanderers". No-one knows where they are wandering in their minds, but, in reality, they are often

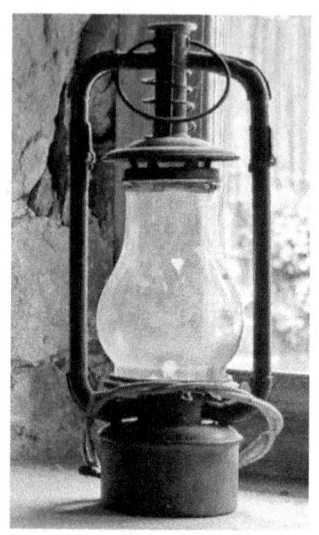

So long as the memory of certain beloved friends lives in my heart, I shall say that life is good.

Helen Keller

wandering towards danger. Sometimes towards their own deaths.

If mum had been able to face reality and all its unpleasantness, she might have realized she had an illness of the mind. Perhaps she might have listened and not become angry when I told her what she was doing, what she was becoming.

Perhaps she might have seen the writing on the wall earlier, when her own mother went through the horrors of Alzheimers disease. My grandmother, also, was a "wanderer". I'm told I was given the job of taking her by the hand and leading her to church. Apparently, I'd introduce her to people thus: "This is my grandmother. She's 60, *and she's still alive!*" But I guess she didn't remember her own age. Each of her five daughters and the remaining son took turns at caring for her, until she went walkabout. When they found her, she would go off to live with one of the others for a few days or weeks.

"Thank God you're here," she'd say to the new carer. "They were trying to kill me, you know."

Oh yes, the writing was on the wall, if only mum had been prepared or able to see it. But now it was too late. Her own summer had drifted into autumn, like a ghost ship drifting in and out of the fog, and time was a merciless tyrant.

#

AUTUMN was so very short for mum. She had slipped into it unwillingly, late in life, preserving her perfect summer for as long as true grit allowed.

Mum and dad came down from Queensland to live with my wife, Judy, and me in Sydney, when dad thought he was dying and when he could no longer watch and protect mum all the time, or catch her when she went walkabout.

The move traumatized and confused them. While house extensions were being hastily completed to accommodate them, they'd sit for hour after hour in straight-backed chairs, not talking, not reading, not watching TV, not doing anything. Just sitting. Glassy eyes staring into the past. Sometimes they'd drift into sleep, sitting stiffly, bolt upright in their chairs, and Judy and I began to realize what lay ahead.

And now mum started something new.

"Where's mum and dad?" she'd ask, looking straight into your soul with those clear, sharp, intelligent eyes. How those eyes confused me. There was never the slightest hint that something was amiss behind them. They were so direct, so challenging.

"Ah, well, mum... don't you remember? Your mum and dad died many years ago. A long time ago. We're in 1999 now... remember?" Then, trying to ease her distress: "They are in heaven now, mum."

She would sit there. Confused. Trying desperately to understand.

"Dead? Mum *and* dad? Dead? Why didn't somebody tell me?"

She'd sit looking at me, trying to work things out. Perhaps it did not help that she had *not* been told of her father's death immediately, because she was busy giving birth to my brother, and she missed his funeral.

"Where's mum and dad?" she'd ask. Again. And again. And again.

Dad, a strong man, would cry and his head would go down and his voice would break, and Judy and I began to develop the fine and frustrating art of distracting mum.

Trying to settle mum and dad into their new section of our home drove *us* to distraction. Before they left Queensland, we had implored them to sell or give

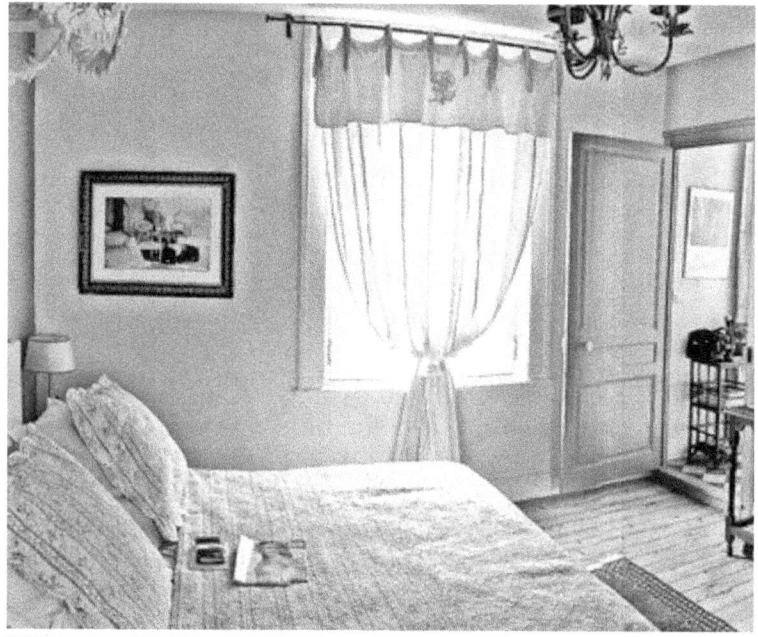

She wanted to fit her whole house into part of ours.

away excess furniture, white goods, clothes they would never wear, tools and utensils they would never use. It's all here, we'd say. But mum was no longer capable of rational thought, so down came about three times as much as we could fit in. Absolute nightmare. Mum would part with nothing. She had about thirty cushions for one lounge suite, for God's sake.

Finally, we had a "garage sale" to sell what we and mum and dad could no longer use. Problem. As we were trying to sell things spread out on our lawn and under our carport, mum would recognize things.

"Oh look," she'd say. "I have one just like that." And she'd whisk that item away and back into the house.

This went on all day. She'd take something away, we'd sneak it back. She'd see it again and take it away. We'd sneak it back. You do learn to be dishonest and duplicitous when dealing with dementia. You have to be. And that's very, very hard when it's your mum, the one who taught you your values in the first place. She looks deep into your eyes, and you know she has always known when you equivocate - but you have to steady yourself, and lie. I've never been good at lying, and I'd pray she didn't notice.

Someday, those who care for a person with Alzheimer's may be faced with what appears to be an insoluble problem. Caregivers may try everything they have been taught, but nothing works. So, they touch the arm of the person with Alzheimer's and speak gently. The caregiver may hug the person with Alzheimer's or give a kiss and tell her that she is loved. One day, if the caregiver is lucky, a revelation occurs. That person learns that the last thing we ever lose is love. Our memories may be gone. But we remember love.

Tim Brennan

But there was no lying to her when dad had his stroke; it happened right in front of her. She refused to move while we tended to him, or when the ambulance arrived, or when the paramedics worked on him.

Finally, she turned to me, tears streaking her face: "Don't let them take him to hospital, will you?"

She had always feared hospitals. When I was eight, she had to have all her teeth removed and she refused to go to hospital. She had them out at home, on the kitchen table. You only went to hospital for one reason, she thought - to die. It was a thought she could never shake loose.

"Don't worry, mum," I lied, again. "We'll just take him to the doctor."

Dad recovered remarkably well (I had always said you couldn't kill him with an axe), but mum never did recover.

Within a month, she had collapsed with her own stroke and slipped deep into Alzheimer's disease - and into her winter years.

I have seen deeply demented
patients weep or shiver
as they listen to music
they have never heard before,
and I think they can
experience the entire
range of feelings
the rest of us can,
and that dementia,
at least at these times,
is no bar to emotional depth.
Once one has seen such
responses, one knows that
there is still a self
to be called upon, even if
music, and only music,
can do the calling.

Oliver Sacks

Winter: The Demon of Dementia

THE spring, summer and autumn of mum's life seemed to go on forever, until the day in her 87th year, when her brain finally closed down and never fully reopened.

Winter fell that day, and fair weather never returned.

Her final two years were spent in two nursing homes and three hospitals, and in a desperate search for a way to go home.

CAMPBELLTOWN HOSPITAL

OLD age should be an estuary that spreads serenely as it empties itself into the sea. But mum came to the sea down a steep, narrow chasm and her rapids crashed and surged until she fell, exhausted, into the deep.

#

MUM's first three months in hospital were a nightmare. She was at times a hostile patient, a lost child who could never find her mother and father, an old lady absolutely bewildered by her surroundings.

She was sometimes extremely hostile. She hit a security guard over the head with a heavy glass jar and staff decided they really had to do something about this tiny little old lady who had extraordinary strength and determination. They could not contain her and started to talk of restraining and sedating her.

She kept thinking she was going to picnics or parties. At one time, she actually did crash a party. Hospital staff were having a farewell party for one of the nurses. As soon as mum walked in and realized it was a party, she naturally thought it was for her.

She sat in a chair in a central location, so that party-goers had to party around her, and she would not budge. The hospital sent for us and by the time we got there, the party was over, but she was still in the chair, sound asleep and set like concrete. I could not prize her out of that chair.

It's amazing how stiff mum became as she got

older. She was always stiff, and cold, her bones so near the surface, so that, if you touched her, you felt the bones, stiff through the skin. There was always that stiffness about her. A rigidity of nature and a physical stiffness that was always a little off-putting. However, as she got older, it became worse, as if she was, indeed, made of stone or concrete.

And this is how we found her on the day of "her" party. We got her back to her room by picking her up, chair and all, with the help of security men. Only when she was back in her room did she wake and, of her own volition, get out of the chair and into bed.

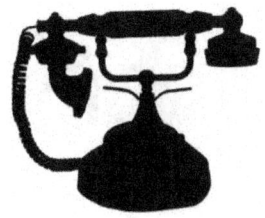

MEMORY is a funny thing. Mum's short-term memory was like the water in a pond. Things would disturb the surface, but then the water would close in again, as if nothing had happened.

Yet her long-term memory, at least for a time, remained intact. Perhaps it was because the events

A friend knows the song in my heart and sings it to me when my memory fails.
Author unknown

It is strange how we hold on to the pieces of the past while we wait for our futures.
Author unknown

remembered had occurred long, long ago in a different world.

And her feelings were all present when needed, as if they were not bundled with memory but stored in a different place.

We would watch her closely, and it appeared that events that happened beneath the surface, deeper in the past, and deeper in the heart, lasted longest.

She fluctuated wildly between old age and childhood, never able to find the words to talk to anyone about it. Always alone with a mind that betrayed her and tormented her.

#

THEY are everywhere. Thieves. I can trust no-one, especially the men. And the school children, of course. Why do their parents allow them to roam this place, stealing everything? And the noise they make.

"No, mum," he says, "there are no school children here, only adults. And I'm sure your clothes are safe. See? Judy has sown your name on each item so everyone will know they are yours."

I laugh and I can taste the bitterness.

"You don't know what goes on here, when you're not here," I say. *"You leave me and go away, and it's dreadful."*

I start to cry. Nobody knows the things they do to you. When you are trapped. Alone. At night. When your mother and father won't come for you.

Judy's talking again.

"Mum, did I tell you Fiona's boy, Sean, is in school now? He loves it - and he looks so good in his school uniform."

Fiona? Sean?

"Oh, yes?" I say. *It will come to me in a minute. What were those names again?*

And the other thing... what was I thinking? It was pretty bad, I know. It will come to me in a minute.

Sometimes they mix me up, the things they say.

AT times in Campbelltown Hospital, she thought she was a member of staff. In particular, she thought she was a cleaner, because nobody could clean the place as well as she could. She would follow the real cleaners around, cleaning up after them.

There was a corridor that ran all around the

rectangular ward and around that corridor ran a railing on both sides. It became mum's obsession to clean that railing, walking around and around and around, polishing it with a cleaning cloth. When we visited, she would complain bitterly that "they" would give her no relief and no staff to help her.

"And the pay is dreadful," she'd say. "I have absolutely no money. No money at all. I can't even go out and do the shopping."

Another time, she was found in the kitchen, washing up a huge pile of crockery and glassware. We very quickly had to get her away from that. Mum's hands shook at the best of times, and these were *not* the best of times.

#

I HATE mirrors. I spend a lot of time staring into the glass, trying to make out who is there. Or why it is me, but not me. Sometimes it looks like me, sometimes the face is familiar, but different.

Sometimes I feel dazed, confused, curious, distressed. Sometimes they all seem to happen at once. I just don't know. I can't work it out. Is it me standing there or someone trying to look like me?

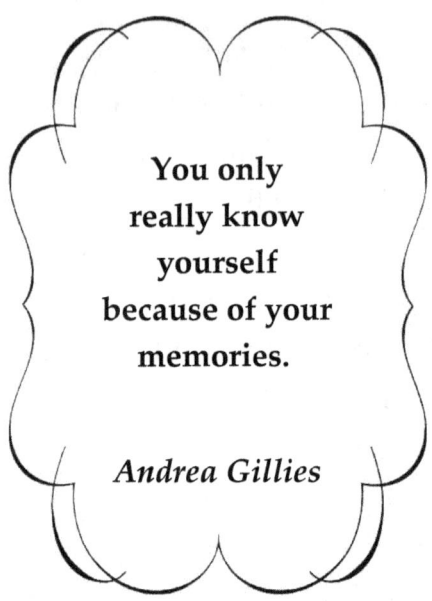

You only really know yourself because of your memories.

Andrea Gillies

Sometimes I think I must be dreaming. She doesn't look like me, not like the real Kathleen. It doesn't feel like me. I am dreaming. Am I?

I get so mixed up I try to only use the mirror if no-one is looking. Sometimes they see me. Sometimes I can't help it; I can feel my face crumble. I am distraught. I know something bad has happened, but I'm not sure what. I just can't stop crying.

And who is that who is watching me? Who is that person in the mirror? Why is she in my mirror? But I cannot ask and I'll just stay away from that mirror. And her.

\#

Mum would lay in her bed, looking out her window and see things that we couldn't see. She'd see, for example, the double decker bus or the tram coming to take her and the rest of the school children to school or to a picnic.

She would see her friends, up in the trees (her ward was two floors up). She'd wave to them and call out and was always disappointed when they ignored her. Sometimes they did shout back, and wave to her, she thought, and she would beam with pleasure.

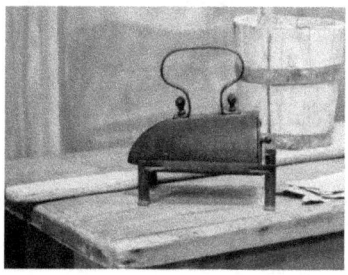

MUM spent her first in-care Christmas in that hospital and the Christmas tree was the bane of her life.

Staff had erected a huge Christmas tree in a corner, thinking it would be a distraction for mum and some of the other patients. The ward had been sealed and locked because mum was a wanderer, so all the patients were basically prisoners in that ward. The tree was something to brighten their days.

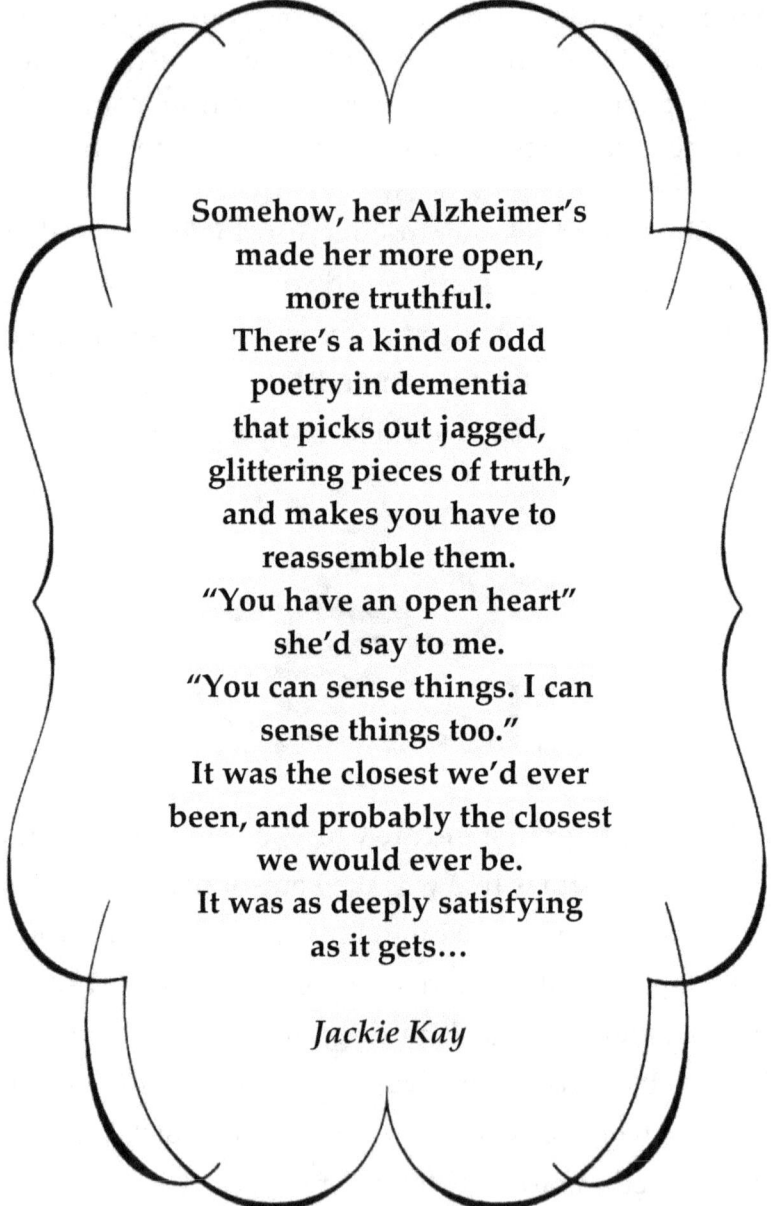

Somehow, her Alzheimer's
made her more open,
more truthful.
There's a kind of odd
poetry in dementia
that picks out jagged,
glittering pieces of truth,
and makes you have to
reassemble them.
"You have an open heart"
she'd say to me.
"You can sense things. I can
sense things too."
It was the closest we'd ever
been, and probably the closest
we would ever be.
It was as deeply satisfying
as it gets...

Jackie Kay

Staff spent several hours decorating that tree. Then, every day, three or four times a day, at least, mum pulled every decoration off and redecorated. She did it because she was convinced someone was coming in after her and "mucking it up". And, anyway, nobody could do it like she could. Nobody could achieve the perfection she could.

And so the first Christmas came and went under a hundred different Christmas trees in mum's ward.

#

LANGUAGE was always difficult for the dementia patients.

Some could not speak at all. Some could manage a phrase or a word or two. Some would start a sentence and forget, part way through, what they were talking about and finish the sentence with another thought, or part thought. Some thought they were speaking, but you couldn't make out a word of it.

This was all brought home early in mum's final illness, through one of the other patients with dementia at Campbelltown Hospital, a man we came to call Paul the Pole (to distinguish him from another

Paul). He was a short man, bald, bandy, perhaps about 60 years of age. He was a Polish-born Australian.

When we met him, he could only speak his native tongue, because he had learnt English later in life and now he had reverted, in his illness, to childhood. No-one was ever able to get him to speak in English or to understand it again.

Later, Paul became one of mum's "family" in Rose House, but, by then, he could not speak at all, nor could he understand what was said to him.

IN the big ward at Campbelltown Hospital, I often strolled around the long corridor with mum. It was usually done to distract her when she became upset and aggressive. We would go for a walk and she would forget, we hoped, what had been on her mind.

Every time we passed a doorway, she would look inside, greet the people there, tell me who they were (though names eluded her) and introduce me. In some doorways, I was Bert, in others Arthur, in some Brian, and in many, she'd have to ask my name. The people inside were her childhood friends, her family, people she knew from church. She couldn't remember names, but it didn't matter. The men were always "that man" (whom she would describe as her brother, or father, or son) and the women were always "Eileen". We have no idea where the name Eileen came from, but, from there on, in three hospitals and two nursing homes, all the women were Eileen.

THE main problem in that ward, apart from her desperation to go home, was mum continually thinking she was hearing her mother and father and her daughter.

One of the strange things about dementia is that patients can think of their parents, who are long gone, and their children, who are now adults with grandchildren, in the same thought or in the same sentence, as all being alive, without noticing anything amiss. They can live in the past and the present at the same time.

Mum could forever hear her mother and father and it distressed her terribly that she could hear them and they refused to come in to see her.

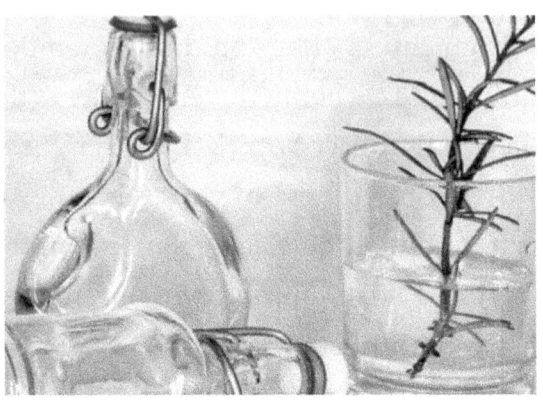

She was continually looking for her mother and father on our walks. One day, she pointed through a doorway and said, "There's dad. Don't disturb him, he's sleeping." It turns out mum had treated the poor man as her father all day. For several hours during the morning, she had sat by his side, holding his hand and talking to him, as if she were a child once more.

Then as we left his room, there was a hint of scandal, or more than a hint of scandal, in her voice. It seems *another woman* had been visiting her father. You can imagine mum's shock. Hers had been an absolutely blameless family in that regard. You only had to ask mum to know that.

"She," said mum, "*She* has been coming and going every day. Every day." Her tone of voice and the way she rolled her eyes told me that her poor mother knew nothing about this disgusting liaison. Mum shook herself, drew her shoulders back and marched off. It was clear that her father, of his own volition, would never, *never*, be involved in a scandal like this. She, *she*, must have seduced the poor man (though mum, of course, would never actually use a wicked word like "seduce").

#

THE other person that mum could never find was her daughter, Diane, my sister. Diane was actually 800 miles away to the north, beyond Brisbane, but every time mum heard a nurse or a patient call out, she thought it was Diane. And again, she was so distressed when Diane "refused" to come in and see her.

Again and again we'd try to explain that Diane was not there, and she would understand. Or seem to. But within minutes, she'd be calling for Diane again and asking us to fetch her.

This went on for hour after hour, day after day, week after week, despite our desperate efforts to break the cycle.

#

AS part of mum's continual agitation and aggressive badgering to get home, she drove us mad with her clothing.

We would lay everything out, organize everything in her wardrobes, and we would come back to visit her next time only to find it was all off the hangers, in her bags and hidden. We emptied the bags and took them away, but she managed to find plastic bags, which were even easier for her to hide, ready to take home.

I used to pretend that I was her butler and nobody else could lay her clothes out as well as I could, and she would agree, not remembering, but assuming I was, indeed, her butler. In that way I could get her clothes, or most of them, hung up or put away again, but it was only temporary and they would be out again next visit. Very often she would not allow me to hang certain items, because she did not want to wear these things in hospital. She wanted me to take them home, ready for her. I would smuggle them back to the wardrobe, but they would be hidden again next time we visited.

Later, there was a problem with other people's clothing, as mum began to hoard these things in her wardrobe. She would find things she thought were hers, and take them. Later again, it extended to photographs. Mum saw photos and thought they were of her family and she would take them and put them up on her shelf. Sometimes she'd hide them in case somebody found them and stole them from her.

This, of course, applied to all the patients, who all had clothing and personal items they thought were theirs, but belonged to someone else. Staff did their best to sort things out, but often could only throw their hands in the air.

THE call from Campbelltown Hospital came through late at night, as these things usually do.

"We can't control your mother. She has become violent. Can you come in?"

Mum had been aggressive previously, and, just the day before, Judy and I had given permission for doctors to sedate her and restrain her when needed. But we had emphasized that only mild sedation would be necessary, because mum reacted badly to strong medications.

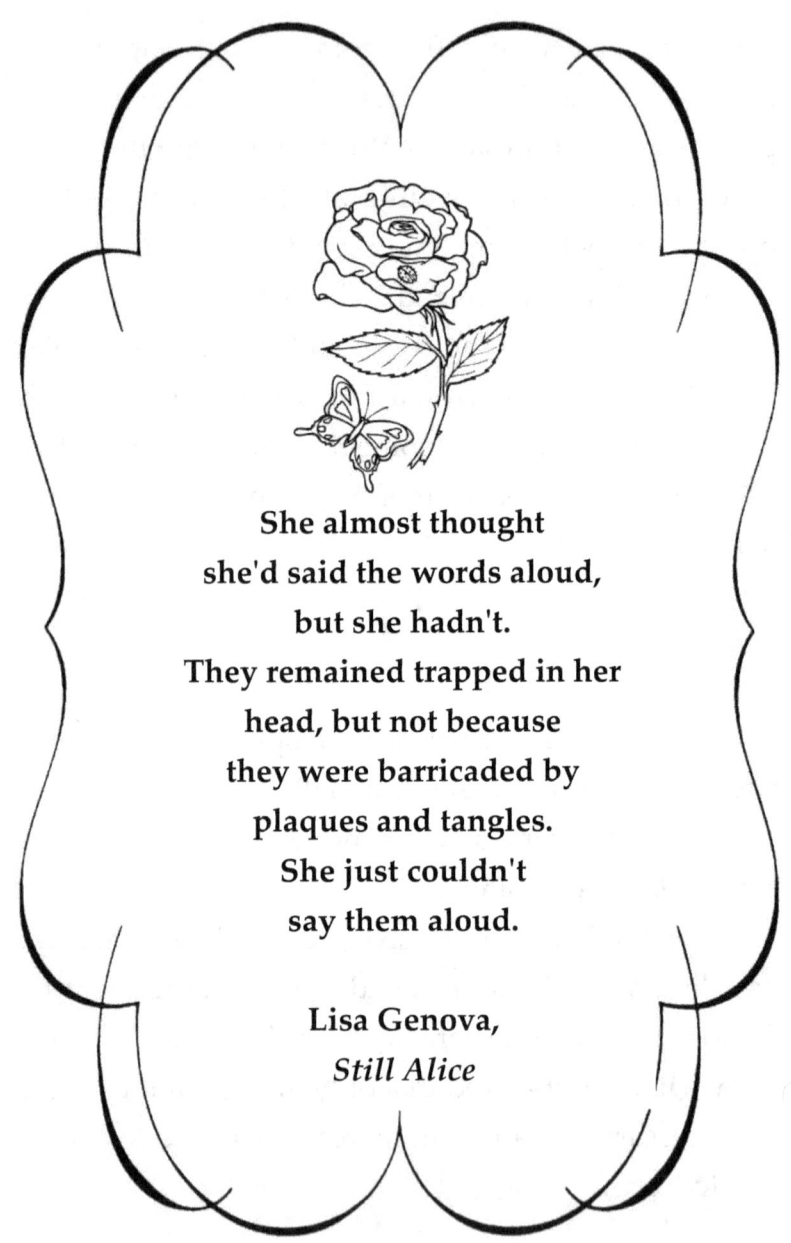

She almost thought
she'd said the words aloud,
but she hadn't.
They remained trapped in her
head, but not because
they were barricaded by
plaques and tangles.
She just couldn't
say them aloud.

Lisa Genova,
Still Alice

The half-hour drive to the hospital took me about fifteen minutes. It must be bad, I thought, if sedation wasn't working. Mum weighed very little dripping wet, but she had amazing strength. However, I had been able to settle her in the past, just over the phone.

When I arrived, the light over her door was flashing and her room was full of people. An alarm was sounding.

I had been, in the past, editor and manager of our city's newspapers and Judy had worked in the hospital for ten years, so I knew a "Code Blue" when I saw one.

I rushed to the doorway and was quickly, roughly, pushed out. Two nurses took me and explained what I already knew. Mum had reacted badly to the sedation and her blood pressure had crashed. She had "gone flat" and collapsed into unconsciousness. Her heart had stopped beating.

There was noise and confusion and rushing all around me, but it was as if I was dreaming. I realized immediately that I could do nothing. I was not feeling anything and time did not exist. At once I could see everything that was happening. The doctors. The equipment. The injection. The thud and jump as they put the disks on mum's frail body and hit her with the charge. In an instant I comprehended all of it, and then time stopped.

But they brought her around. She had died and now lived again. And I wondered why.

I sat with her, holding her bony hand while she slept. Surely God had decided it was time, but the doctors had vetoed the decision.

At what stage should life end? Now that they had brought her back, what did the future hold? More suffering? Loss of dignity? The agony of despair?

The answers were beyond me.

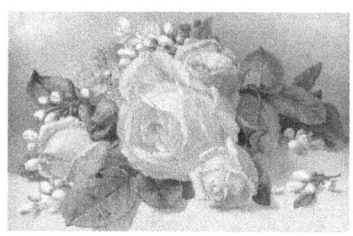

THE thing that finally convinced dad that we could not look after mum at home was a fall she took in Campbelltown Hospital.

She wanted to go to the toilet and was too frail to take herself. There were a few emergencies in the ward and there were no nursing staff available, so I took her. I assumed it might be an "emergency" for her because she had become incontinent and was not aware, usually, of her need for the toilet until the last minute.

I had a bad back and legs. I was stiff. I had no strength. I didn't know at the time that I had a condition called Fibromyalgia, apart from the spinal problems, and I attempted to get mum to the toilet, look after her clothing, sit her down on the toilet and hold her there. As she was sitting, she twisted. In the process of twisting, she fell and slipped away from me. I weighed twice what she did, but I could not hold her.

She fell down between the toilet and the wall, and, for her, it was hilarious. She giggled as if she was a schoolgirl, whereas she would have been horrified if she had been truly aware of her circumstances.

I was unable to lift her. I was in severe pain, just trying to stop her slipping further. I shouted for dad to get help and the nursing staff were able to get her up and take care of her.

On the way home from the hospital, dad was silent for a while, then admitted, for the first time, that there was no way we could look after mum at home. He had spoken the words before, but did not truly believe them, always hoping against hope that we could bring her home.

"There's a word for it," she
told me, "in French,
for when you have a lingering
impression of something
having passed by.
Sillage.
I always think of it when a
firework explodes and lights
up the smoke from
the ones before it."
"That's a terrible word," I
teased. "It's like an excuse for
holding onto the past."
"Well, I think it's beautiful.
A word for remembering
small moments
destined to be lost."

Robyn Schneider

However, apart from the wandering, she needed continual medical and physical care. That was now abundantly clear. It's one thing for medical staff to tell you, another thing to see it for yourself. For dad, it was the final recognition of mum's true state.

BUT we didn't just have to worry about mum, and about dad's reaction to her illness. Our greatest fears came from the Australian Federal Government's Aged Care Assessment Team (ACAT).

It was ACAT's task to assess people for the various levels of nursing care. These wonderful souls wanted to put mum into a mental institution while she waited for a place in a secure nursing home.

It was their job to find the nursing home place, but they were not just incompetent, they made no effort whatsoever.

There was no way mum was going into a mental institution. No way. But how to stop the institutional steamroller?

Judy and I attacked on a number of fronts. We first took legal action to take control of mum's finances.

Without money, no nursing home could accept mum, so we effectively stopped her being placed in an unsuitable place or one that we couldn't visit. (This was all with dad's approval).

Next, we tied up the hospital bureaucracy and the government bureaucracy (which administered the hospital system) with paperwork. Bureaucracies are unable to operate in a flood of paper. This meant they were unable to transfer mum to a mental institution. Mum was effectively locked into her hospital ward, as comfortable a place as we could hope for, until a suitable nursing home place was found.

I was well equipped to look after these first two steps, but I was really struggling emotionally with the third step - finding mum a suitable place. Demand for nursing home places greatly outstripped supply at that time and it was a harrowing experience.

Thank God I had Judy. I found some vacancies, but I wouldn't put mum in them. She was aware enough of her circumstances for their condition to have broken her heart. But Judy was marvelous. She persisted on the phone until she found a place at Pendle Hill, a Sydney suburb, which was ideal for mum, though difficult for us to visit. Mum's needs came first.

We moved mum, then Judy and I turned our attention to ACAT. We didn't want anyone else to have to go through what we went through. The upshot was that the entire team was dismissed and a new team appointed. We were not overjoyed at this result, but our old folk deserve better, and they can't fight for themselves.

Later, Judy was to find another place for mum, after she collapsed and needed high level nursing care that Pendle Hill could not provide. I wish mum had been able to understand what Judy had done for her.

CHURCH OF CHRIST NURSING HOME,
PENDLE HILL

THE past became an uncontrollable kaleidoscope that turned and jumbled its light and shadow every time a thought dropped into place. A thousand images jostled for prominence in a crazy tumble of living memories. Parents, sisters, brothers, relatives, school friends, church friends, neighbours, family - some long dead, others long forgotten in reality hours - all slipped in and out of view like a shifting, pitching mosaic.

Focus on this, and it fled into hiding; focus on that,

Looking at my reflection, in the window opposite, hollow and translucent, I see a woman disappearing. It would help if I looked like that in real life – if the more the disease advanced, the more 'see-through' I became until, eventually, I would be just a wisp of a ghost. How much more convenient it would be, how much easier for everyone, including me, if my body just melted away along with my mind. Then we'd all know where we were, literally and metaphysically."

Rowan Coleman

and it dissolved into something, someone else.

Images slipped so easily out of grasp. A thousand faces, all without names, pitched and tossed as on a storm-wracked sea.

Reality and illusion played havoc on a fragile mind. Joy and sorrow swamped a brittle heart.

It was like living in a perpetual fog - watching and waiting for things to reveal themselves and form into blurs of memories.

WHO is this who comes? Is this someone I know? Could that be Bert? Yes, and that's Gladys with him, isn't it? Who is that? I'll smile. It's probably them. I'll straighten up. Look at them. Smile.

They walk past. They are going to someone else. They're sitting down with them. Why are they doing that? Can't they see me here? Don't they know me? I'm sure I know them. Maybe I don't. Maybe they just look like my family.

Why don't my family ever visit me? Why am I the only one who never has a visitor? Why am I the only one who is so lonely? Dear Lord, why am I the only one all alone?

I won't let them see me cry.

Lord, the ache in my chest. I can't breathe. But I won't let them see me cry.

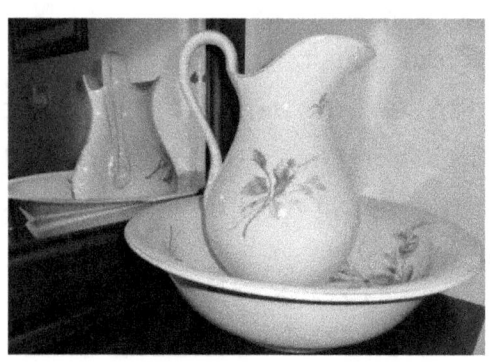

THERE was a secret side to mum that nobody ever managed to penetrate. Not even dad.

She was a creator of illusions that people saw as realities, but were not. She even deceived *herself* into believing things were true that were not.

In these illusions, the real Kathleen was nowhere to be seen. She created a fantasy world that rejected reality and tended to what might have been, or, more to the point, what *should* have been. She pushed aside disturbing thoughts, but she never managed to truly let go of anger, hatred, resentment. Every now and then, the cauldron would boil over and out it would all spill.

But this happened only rarely. Mum's control was remarkable. Usually, and until very late in life, she showed no feelings or emotions. I'm sure that, to her way of thinking, this would indicate a lack of control.

#

LIFE became a kind of memory dance - one step sideways, two steps back, towards the past, towards youth and childhood.

But, for every moment of seeing youth through the looking-glass of illusive memory, there was a corresponding moment of seeing age through a mirror of reality.

Every bathroom had such a mirror. Every nurse, every visitor spoke such reality.

Life had become a series of broken dreams.

#

I NOTICE the bedspread is crooked. It's that housemaid. You can't get good help... I'll have to do it myself.

Big job. Big bed spread. I've seen this pattern and these

Memories were the only things that made aging bearable, a way of reverting to better, simpler days.

Andrea Lochen

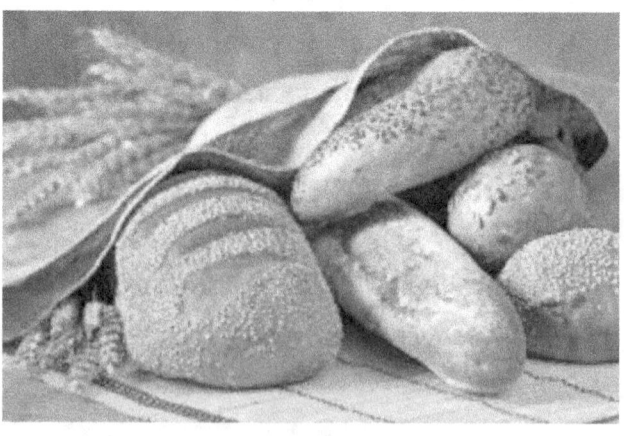

folds before. Where? Where did I see them?

Straighten it out a bit. Hard to get it just right. Fix this bit and that bit is crooked. Fix that, and this is all wrong.

Ah, now I see the other blanket, but it's spread out on the ground. Sounds from another time, another place, begin to whisper to me. The whispering of yesteryear.

I listen. Laughter. Voices. It's a picnic. Who's there? I hear Gladys. And Arthur. Trust Arthur to be drinking beer. He'll cop it if mum sees him.

Ah, there are the others. There's Vida and Amy and Elsie. Mum's pouring cordials. Here comes dad and Bert with the kindling. They'll have the barbecue going in no time.

"What are you doing with that bedspread, Kathleen? Come on, I'll fix it. Let's go, it's time for lunch. Come on, Kathleen. Let's go. Let's go now."

The whispering stops.

I WALK into the ward, into mum's room, and I can see immediately it's going to be a difficult visit. They all were, in one way or another, but sometimes mum was particularly upset.

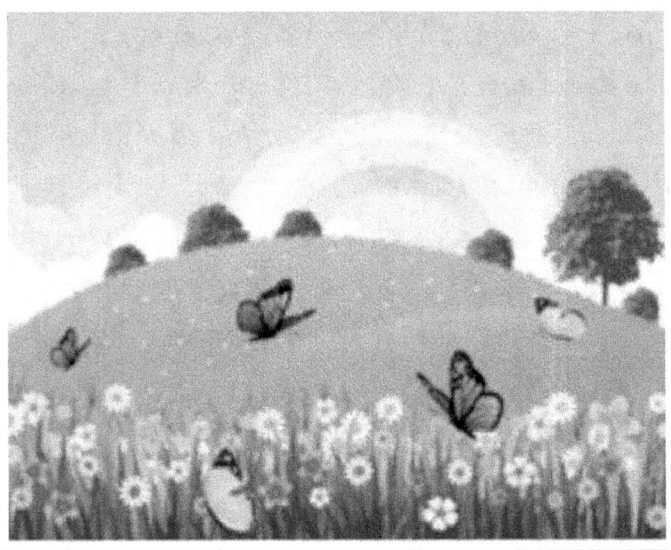

A day close to perfection.

"What's wrong, mum?" I ask.

"I don't want to go to school anymore," she says. "I've had enough. I can't do that arithmetic any more. I'm not going. That's all there is to it. I'm not going."

"There's no need for you to go to school, mum," I say. "Heck, I reckon you know it all by now, anyway. You've been going for a long time, haven't you? I'll talk to the nuns. I'm sure you won't have to go at all."

And she begins to settle and she sits for a while. Then she stiffens.

"I don't want to go to school anymore," she says. "And I will not go. You'll see. I will not go."

And over and over and over it we go.

THERE is a day that stands out, a day closer to perfection than I ever expected to see again in times of dementia.

We are in the courtyard of the nursing home on a morning of glorious sunshine and dizzying warmth. Gardens bloom on all sides, each competing for attention with the crispness of spring, the dazzle of colour and the heady richness of perfume. Bees buzz. Birds sing in their cage.

A winding path leads from the nursing home door around the garden and back again to the door. By the time patients stroll its length, they think they've had an adventure and have arrived home again.

I sit at the garden table with mum, dad and Judy, who is keeping mum occupied by cleaning and trimming her nails. Other patients come and go, thinking they and we are all family. As, I guess, we are.

We soak up the sun and talk of yesterdays that mum might remember. We switch to the present if the past makes her sad, or back to the past if the present brings a tear. Switching back and forth this way, we keep mum mostly happy.

And that is what makes the morning so special. Her smile. The laughter in her eyes. Even if her speech is a jumble, her heart is light. She is young again. And beautiful.

It is a morning to fill the heart.

As we are leaving, mum touches my arm. "Thanks for coming to my party," she says.

Then she hesitates. "I think I should know you, shouldn't I?"

#

IN all her desperation to get home, in the end, mum couldn't tell you where home was. She'd ask, "Where are we living now?" and she couldn't remember the last place she lived.

The only place she could remember from time to time was Campsie, the suburb of Sydney where she grew up. But whether or not she could remember where home was, there was always the restless, sad, despairing search for it.

I WALK down the corridor, looking in every nook and cranny. I hear noises, but, when I spin around, they are gone. They are getting closer. I try to get help, but they all just smile and say something and walk away. For God's sake...

They are trying to kill me. Can't anyone understand?

I slip quietly into my room. I see nobody, but I know they're here. I look in the cupboards and wardrobes. Nothing. I look under the bed. Nothing.

But I hear them. They are here. I know it - and they are going to kill me.

My heart is beating so fast and the pain in my chest is awful. I'll get into bed and hide under the sheets. Be very quiet. Say my prayers.

Ah, that's better. I didn't realize I was so tired. I might have a little nap and then have a cup of tea.

Perhaps the family will come this afternoon. Yes, that would be lovely. It is a lovely day for visitors.

MUM was always a remote kind of person. Until late in life, I never realized that neither mum nor dad ever played with me as a child. I suppose, when it didn't happen, I didn't expect it to happen.

I have vivid recollections of childhood, but not one of either of them ever playing with a ball, pushing a swing or doing anything with me, apart from going shopping or doing other adult things. Perhaps that's just the way things were, back then.

Although mum's children were her whole universe, she was never able to grow close to them. It never occurred to me, for example, that I could confide in mum, either as a child or as an adult.

She was a rigid woman who had to keep control of everything and everyone around her (and I, unfortunately, would not be controlled). She was stiff in spirit and stiff physically. I remember her cold, stiff hands. Not just in her illness, but for many years. And she always felt the cold, dressing in layer upon layer of clothing.

Even her kiss was cold. Not that I ever thought her heart was cold, her lips were. And where once she was sprightly, in the winter of her years she was reduced to the small, stiff steps they call *marche à petit pas*.

An enduring memory was mum's slow shuffle down the corridor of the nursing home, supported by a nurse, who was distracting her while I "escaped". It was always very difficult to get away from mum. She was usually in tears and very distressed. She wanted desperately to go home. She would cry. She would become rigid. She would become aggressive. She would cling to you as you tried to leave.

One day, when I was visiting on my own and staff

were occupied with other patients, I had particular difficulty. Usually we visited at least in pairs to make the visiting, and the leaving, easier.

When the time came to leave, mum would not leave me. I tried to distract her, or to leave her in her room, or to take her to sit with other patients - all to no avail. I was on my walking stick and mum could keep up with me - it was one of her better, more mobile days. But time was against me and I had to leave.

The doors at Rose House closed automatically and could only be opened by keying in a code. Visitors were given the code freely because patients were not capable of remembering it.

I walked to the door, with mum clinging to me. I keyed in the code, with mum watching closely. I pushed the door open, enough for me to slide out. At the same time, I held mum away and told her to step back and watch out, the door was dangerous.

I slipped out and the door closed and locked itself. It was one of my worst moments in two years of visiting. I think it was the most horrible thing I ever did to her. It all happened so fast, but her face was only inches from the door and I still had time to see the look of anticipation on her face turn to a crumbling sadness.

I can see that face still, and will see it until the day I die.

SHE was no wombat, hiding from life in a dark borough. She always needed light.

Her butterfly mind was in constant flight from darkness to light, from complexity to simplicity, from strangers to childhood friends, from bitterness to contentment, from shadow to sunburst.

She was the butterfly that fluttered brightly around the light until, one day, she hovered too close and fluttered no more.

She had never read the story of Icarus. And nothing would have changed if she had.

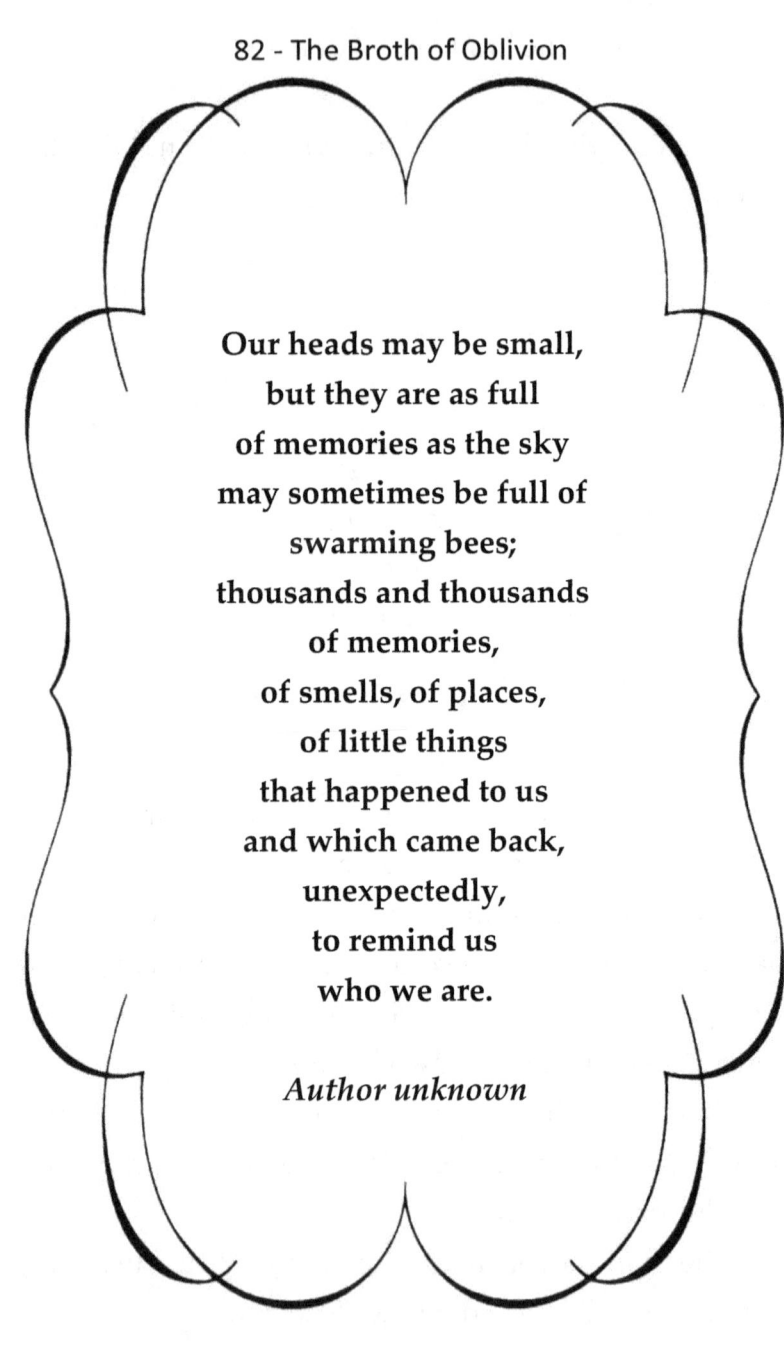

Our heads may be small,
but they are as full
of memories as the sky
may sometimes be full of
swarming bees;
thousands and thousands
of memories,
of smells, of places,
of little things
that happened to us
and which came back,
unexpectedly,
to remind us
who we are.

Author unknown

WESTMEAD HOSPITAL

WE got the call from the Pendle Hill Nursing Home to say that mum had collapsed and had been taken to Westmead Hospital. She had taken a fall out of bed the week before and, as far as the doctors could tell, she was bruised, but OK. But then came the collapse.

We rushed the 45-minute drive to the Emergency Ward and found doctors and nurses hovering around, attending to her. She looked so frail and weak. I wondered how on earth she would survive.

And then came the choice. I was not expecting it.

A young female doctor (I say "female" because women seem to have better bedside manners than their male counterparts) took me aside and said they needed a decision. She took things very slowly.

The gist of it was that, if mum collapsed or there was a deterioration in her condition, should medical staff take drastic and possibly intrusive measures if necessary and do everything to revive her, or should they treat her conservatively and make her comfortable and free of pain?

Immediate thoughts of Campbelltown Hospital flashed into my mind.

The decision was easy, but having to make it was a shock. I was just stunned. I could see no point whatsoever in prolonging mum's agony and I told the doctor that treatment should be conservative, that they should make her comfortable, take away any pain and let nature take its course. The doctor was pleased, because it was the decision they were hoping for, but it was a decision I had to make, not them.

I still can feel that shock when I think of it now, the shock of having to make such a choice about my mother.

MUM's religion had been very important to her throughout her life. I mentioned earlier that neither the Pope nor the Queen ever made it into mum's lounge room, but, on reflection, priests sometimes did. They were, after all, somewhat above royalty.

We had the priests to mum twice during her final illness, and we know they visited a number of times when we weren't there.

The first time was in Westmead Hospital, after mum collapsed. The nursing staff had already called

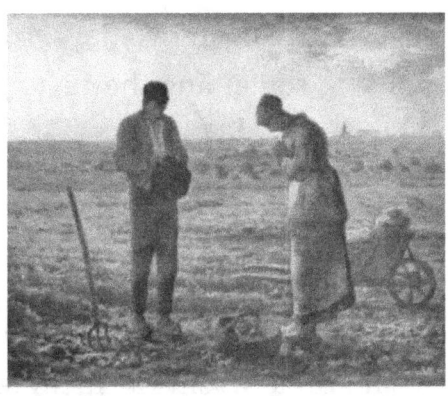

the priest when we asked if he could come. When he arrived, mum was in a very confused and dazed state, but, as soon as we said the priest was there, she seemed to grow still and focus on him.

But then the confusion returned. This priest looked for all the world like an orthodox Jewish rabbi, not the Catholic priest mum was expecting. The full beard, an accent, black suit, white shirt. Mum watched him very, very warily.

The second time was when mum was very frail in Carrington Nursing Home and her heart was playing up. Nursing staff said that she may not have long to live and we called the priest. As soon as he came, mum was again still, focused and watchful.

At the end, when he gave her the Blessing of the Sick, she said, "Thank you, Father." These were the first words she had spoken in two days.

Her religion was something she never truly forgot.

ROSE HOUSE - CARRINGTON NURSING HOME, CAMDEN

MUM liked to think she was the queen of her surroundings. It came from a lifetime of being dominant, of wanting to control her universe.

In the nursing home, people would sit wherever they could find a seat, and usually drop off to sleep. The seats were mostly comfortable lounge chairs and people would just plop. But mum sat on a hard, straight-backed chair in the corner of the living room, and this was her place always.

From here, she could survey her domain. She could sit there and watch everything that went on, for hour after hour. It was as close as she could get to controlling everything. Of course, she, too, slept for much of the time. How she slept in a straight-backed chair, I'll never know, but I'm quite sure she thought it was her throne, and hers alone.

#

The bee fertilizes the flower it robs of nectar. When God took mum's memory away, He fertilized her into a kind of reverse growth, in which she grew from stiffness and the reserve of old age, through various stages of life, to the innocence of childhood.

And, yes, it *was* growth. As the overgrowth and the burden of the mature woman were pruned away, the beauty of the child was revealed, though with beauty and youth come vulnerability and susceptibility to the cruelty of life.

#

WHO is this who stops to laugh and chat and hold my hand? I think I should know her, but her name escapes me. I think it's Eileen.

What a joy she is to ignore the strange things coming out of my mouth. What a delight it is to trust someone like this.

The laugh comes out before I even realize how happy I am.

#

Alzheimer's ...
it is a barren
disease, as
empty and
lifeless as a
desert. It is a
thief of hearts
and souls and
memories.
Nicholas Sparks

Memories
are all
that we
really
own.
*Elias
Lieberman*

HER tears fell on hollow cheeks as she looked at me, again, and asked, "Why did mum and dad leave me here? Why won't they come for me?"

Her eyes, so sharp, looked directly into my soul. How could I lie to her? How could I tell her the truth?

WHEN she became stubborn and dug in her heels and refused to obey an instruction, she could neither articulate her reason nor formulate one.

One is not bad at such times; how can you be bad, when you stubbornly refuse to do what you feel, somehow, is wrong?

TIME is all out of kilter. There is only the present to live in, yet she is not in it. Living in the past was once abhorrent to her; but what can she do now, if only the past seems real? Does this not make the past more precious? Something to cling to?

Would you not grasp this treasure to fill the void

left by an empty present? Would it not be a natural thing to slip into the past and remain there, safe and secure? Until someone brought you back again. To the present. To cruel reality.

HELL is not a place of blazing heat. Hell is a place of lost thought. *That* is torture. When thought is lost, so is hope.

How can we live without hope? How can we live without reaching towards something, and expecting it, or at least wishing for it? But, when you are lost in a world of the past, and cannot focus on the present, let alone the future, of what use is hope? And without use, hope atrophies and dies.

At such times, the natural tendency of all living things to strive for the fulfilment of their yearnings dies. No longer is there that quest for satisfaction in the human breast. Without hope, how can there be an expectation of good? Without hope, despair thrives.

Dante had his hell. Jesus had his Gethsemane. Mum had both. She had lost her way to the future. And she had lost her way home.

#

WE think with our memory. Faulty memory breeds confusion and destroys thought. Without thought, there is no impulse, no quickening of the heart.

But somewhere deep inside, there is the spirit, and mum's spirit would not be chained.

At times, she seemed to know more of her condition than at others, and, when she saw the future with clearer eyes, she fought as Dylan Thomas advised: she "did not go gentle into that good night".

She seemed to instinctively feel she "should burn and rage at close of day; rage, rage, against the dying of the light".

CAMDEN HOSPITAL

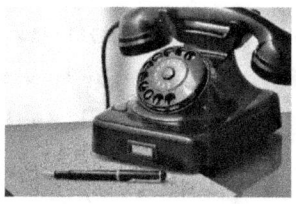

WE lived in dreaded anticipation of a phone call from the nursing home, Rose House, and it came soon enough. Mum had collapsed and had been taken to

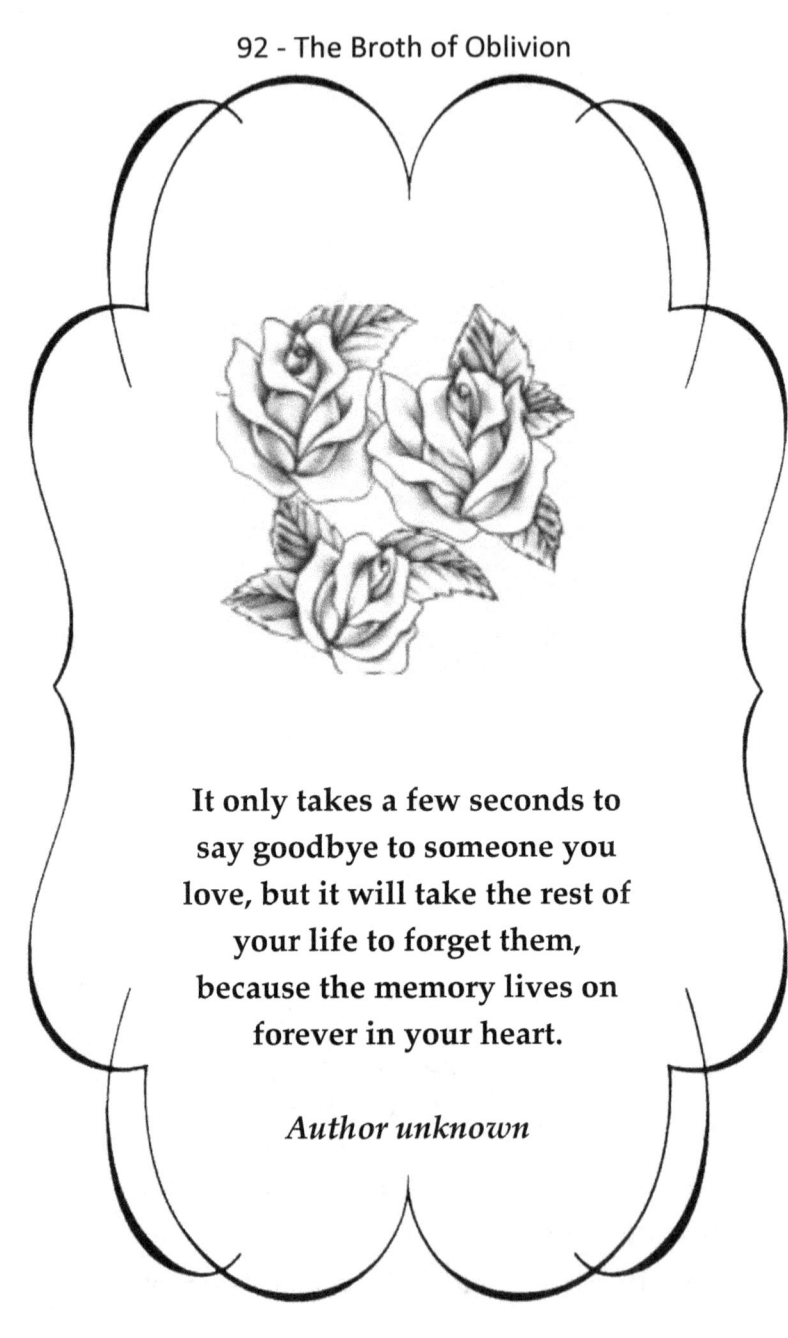

It only takes a few seconds to
say goodbye to someone you
love, but it will take the rest of
your life to forget them,
because the memory lives on
forever in your heart.

Author unknown

Camden Hospital. Judy and I rushed there. I called my brother, Terry, who came immediately. My son, Michael, was also in Sydney, and reached mum first.

We found mum in an observation ward with, perhaps, fifteen other patients. She was very confused.

She understood who Michael was. He had patiently explained who he was, over and over, and she remembered, or thought she remembered him. But she could not understand why she was there. She felt no pain and could not understand why she was in hospital.

But the big problem, the big disturbance for us, when we arrived at the hospital, was to find the way staff treated elderly patients. Mum had on a hospital gown, which hides nothing at the best of times, and she wore nothing else.

No underpants. Nothing. And she was conscious of it. She knew she had no pants on. She kept asking me for them, whispering to me, "Can you get my pants, they're in the drawer." But the drawer was not there. The drawer was back at the nursing home. The pants she had worn to hospital had been soiled and thrown out.

We spoke to the doctors and found that this was

how they treated all elderly people because many had some degree of incontinence. We were disgusted and told them so. Surely there was a solution for people in such a state - disposable pants. This solution worked at home and in nursing homes; why not hospital?

Mum did not stay in the hospital long. I explained the decision I had made in Westmead Hospital about conservative care and told the Camden doctors to mark mum's records with a similar notation. That changed the attitude of the doctors. They observed her for some time, gave her medication and she was allowed to go back to the nursing home.

Back there we discussed the lack of dignity at the hospital. Nursing staff there knew of the hospital policy and were as unhappy with it as we were. We arranged that, was far as possible (and given my instructions for conservative treatment), mum would henceforth be cared for at the nursing home, with the help of the visiting doctor, rather than go to hospital.

Even today, I can still feel mum's horror at the loss of dignity at that hospital. She had always been so proper, but there she was treated as if she had no feelings whatsoever, no importance whatsoever, no humanity.

BACK AT ROSE HOUSE

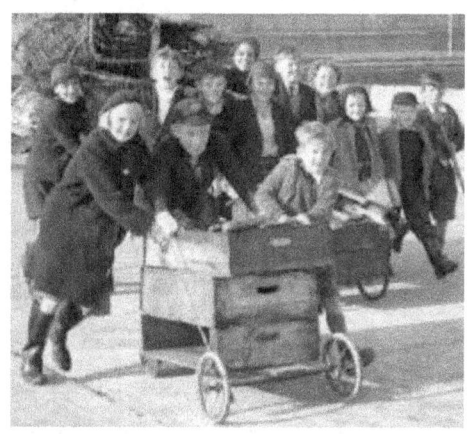

WHEN she closed her eyes and lost herself to the world, she found herself playing in the schoolyard, struggling with an arithmetic lesson, sitting in church with childhood friends, with brothers and sisters, mother and father.

The flame of life was burning low, but sparked whenever she became a child again. And did not the nuns of childhood say that one must become as a child again to enter heaven?

#

SHE heard a different drummer and listened to the beat he made. Her hearing was acute, and she could hear the music though it was far off, or not there at all.

She could hear her parents and her daughter when they were not there. And, for a great deal of the time, she could hear Judy. Judy is cheerful, optimistic, full of life, and every time mum heard someone laugh, she'd laugh herself and say, "There's Judy now." Even if Judy was sitting beside her at the time, perhaps rubbing cream into her dry skin or checking the condition of her legs. (I think it said a great deal that mum could remember Judy's name more often than any other.)

In times like these, when her hearing played tricks on her, mum was in a world much safer and happier than the shadow world she half remembered, the world of reality.

Ah, what a great relief it is, what an inexpressible comfort, to find companionship. To sit with someone who cannot get out of the mouth what is drifting in the mind - and to know it does not matter what strange words come out of my own

mouth. Or whether any words come out at all.

Just to sit with no words and let the mind drift. So peaceful. So sublime.

Sometimes I can only say what I mean when I am silent.

#

A NURSE comes by. She looks at mum. She looks at me.

"If the Good Lord were to tell you He must take away all but one of your blessings," she said, "which would you choose to keep?"

I could find no answer.

"What about memory?" she said. "Without memory, are not most of the other blessings gone? What can withstand the loss of memory?"

Again, I could find no answer.

#

I'M self-taught in history, never having studied it at school (I was never given the option). But I think now of the king of the Greek gods, Zeus. Strange what you think of when you think of memory, but there is a connection.

Zeus was, let's say, a bit of a philanderer. He spent his days and nights seducing, often with deception, the most beautiful women of heaven and earth. But there was one goddess who attracted more of his attentions than any other - Mnemosyne, the goddess of memory.

I shouldn't mention this in polite company, but Zeus once spent nine days and nights making passionate love to Mnemosyne. The result was the birth of the nine muses, each a goddess of a particular art.

The ninth muse was Melpomene, the goddess of tragedy.

And so, I thought, tragedy flows naturally from memory, especially when memory is lost.

IF we lose our memory, forget how we are expected to live, is not our true nature revealed? If you do not comprehend that others can see you, that society expects certain standards from you, will not your true character reveal itself?

In the world of dementia, we reap what we have sown. And what we reap in dementia can surprise and even shock those close to us, because things are revealed that were meant to be concealed.

In dementia, shame has no hiding place.

I HAVE to hide things. They are all thieves here. They take everything.

Sometimes, when I hide things, I find things. I think they steal things and hide them. But I'm too clever for them.

I'll roll up these dirty panties. This really is filthy. How did this happen? I'll put them down the back in this drawer. They'll never know. Roll them up tight. Cover them up.

What's this? Chocolates? These are my chocolates. They must have stolen them and hidden them. I'll hide them again. They won't get them this time.

Ah, there's my purse. They took all my money. Stole it and hid the purse. I'll just push it under the clothes here. They'll never find it.

Look out. Someone's coming. Pretend to do something. Smile so they won't know what I'm doing.

What am *I doing? It'll come to me in a minute.*

#

THIS was a human being, once elegant and articulate, now in soiled clothes, wallowing helplessly in a sea of forgetfulness. And yet, in her bearing, in her essence, dignity's straight back lived on.

She was both heart-wrenchingly strong and pitifully weak.

The paradox of great strength wedded to a child's tenderness, of steel and velvet, of storm and contentment, was a combination that constantly surprised and confused those around her.

#

DAD had been a problem for us since the day mum first went to hospital. He wanted to be with her more often than we could physically or emotionally or practically take him. And, when he was with her, he upset her. Not intentionally, of course, but the result of every visit was the same.

He would sit with his face not six inches from hers. They would look at each other and, for a short time, the look on their faces was beautiful. Then mum's chin would quiver and she'd start to cry and the aggression would soon follow. She didn't know who this man was. She wanted to go home.

Dad would pick at sores on her face or arms, trying to help her, but it always distressed her. He'd point out how a sore had become worse or how her hair needed cutting (you'd think he'd know better than to go down that path!). Once he was walking behind her and trying to brush dirt off her pants. It was not dirt; mum had been incontinent.

Dad always managed to say the wrong thing (although we were all guilty of that from time to time). He was forever bringing up things that we were doing or things that were happening at home - and you know what that led to: more tears and anguish for home.

He was very frail himself by now and he collapsed on one of our visits. We bought him a wheelchair and this helped. I was able to keep him in the wheelchair at Rose House, and keep him at a reasonable distance from mum, so that he was not in her face, or able to touch her and upset her. Judy always helped by keeping mum occupied, with nails, or skin or hair, and doing it in such a way that dad did not get too close.

The doctors and nursing staff didn't want dad to

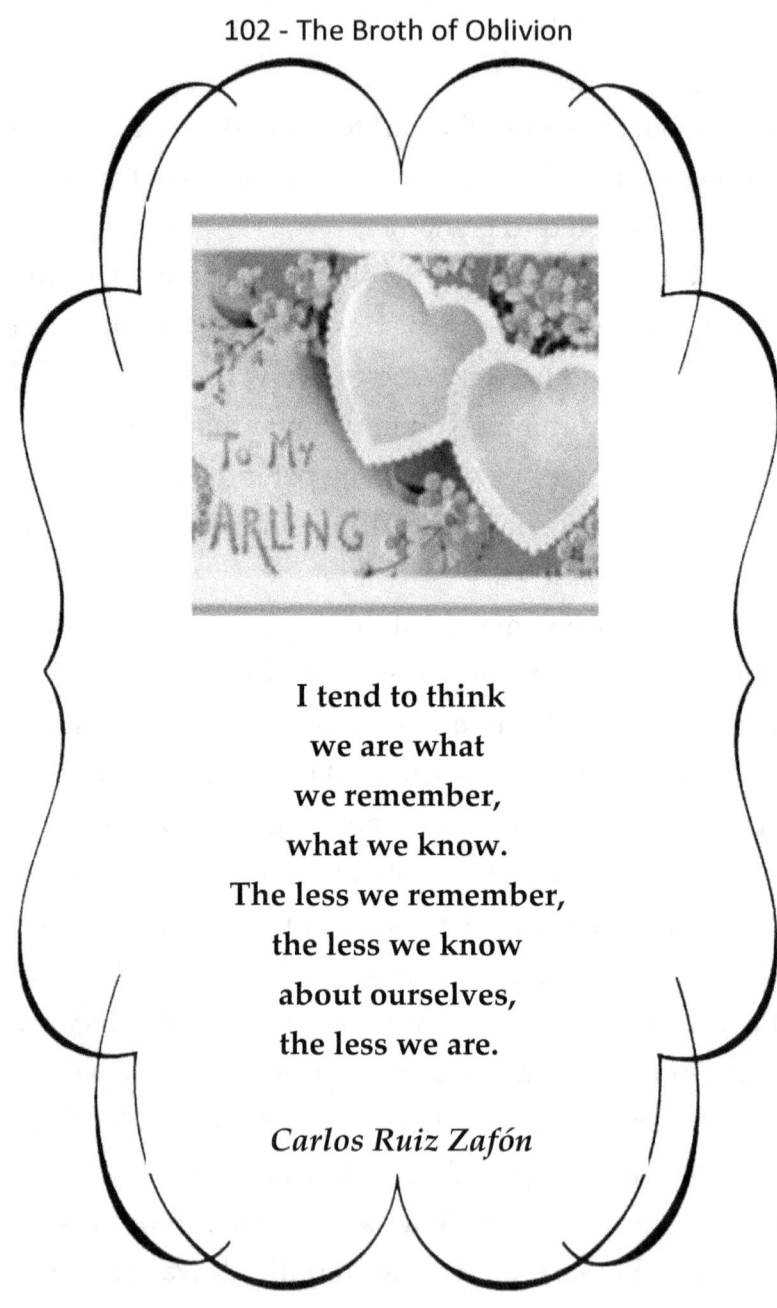

I tend to think
we are what
we remember,
what we know.
The less we remember,
the less we know
about ourselves,
the less we are.

Carlos Ruiz Zafón

visit at all, because it was not good for either mum or dad. His doctor asked him not to visit and said it would be best for mum if he didn't, thinking this would deter him. The nursing staff tried to dissuade him. But he was mule-headed. He could not see how he was hurting mum and he didn't care about himself.

Visiting mum was always hard. Going with dad made it that much harder - not just physically because I had to assemble the wheelchair and push him, but also emotionally. Judy and I were always wrung out after a visit and I was always in considerable pain from pushing the chair.

Dad would not want to eat afterwards. He would cry himself to sleep and sleep for the rest of the day and night. Sometimes, Judy and I wished we could do the same.

#

I KNOW I've asked him before because of the eyes. His eyes betray his lies. Different lies at different times, but still lies. I can't remember the lies, but there were many. I ask him anyway:

"Why do you keep me here? Why don't you let me out?

Why do you hate me? Why..." and I can't stop the tears from falling.

But I'm determined to see his lie, and I watch his eyes. I look into his eyes very deeply, trying to concentrate, but it's happened again. I've forgotten what I asked him.

But I keep staring into his eyes, and, ah yes, they betray him again.

He puts on a hurt look. Looks away and back again. Even has a tear there, but I know it's part of the lie.

"Mum, we can't do anything while you're sick. We have to wait for the doctors to give the all-clear."

That sick business again. Lies. I feel the rage rise up and stiffen me and shake me.

"I am not sick. I haven't been sick for ages. It's an excuse. You hate me and want to lock me away, just like the rest of them. No-one likes me. You all hate me."

I can't look at him anymore. I have these big sobs racking my chest, making me shake. But I can't remember why the sadness is like a vice around my heart.

"Mum, you know that's not true. I wouldn't be here if I didn't love you. Everyone here cares about you. Nobody hates you. How could I hate you?"

Ah, wiping his eyes. Trying to hide his lies.

"Then why am I here? What is this place? A hospital?

Why don't you take me home? I'll never go home again will I? You're trying to keep me locked up here. I hate it here. I'll break out of here. You'll see."

I look into his eyes and remember something else.

"Have you seen mum? I can hear her. She's here, but she won't come to see me. Why won't she come to see me?"

He's much quieter now, and he's looking at the floor.

"Mum," he says, softly, "your mother died a long time ago, remember? Many years ago. She's in heaven now. Remember?"

The fist around my heart becomes cold and tight. What did he say? What nonsense. What did he say? I can't remember what he's been saying. What's happening?

Something bad must have happened because I have such wretched sadness aching inside, and he's kissing me and he's leaving. He doesn't seem able to talk. He's leaving.

"Come on, Kathleen," says the girl. "Let's go to lunch. Isn't it a lovely day? Let's have something to eat."

She has her arm around me and we walk towards the restaurant. Or is it the dining room? She's so cheerful.

"Look at those beautiful carnations. Have you ever seen anything so lovely?"

"No," I say, "My son brought them. He never forgets."

It is a lovely day. I hold on to my friend. Such a lovely

day. I feel like singing. Almost like singing, but I giggle instead with my friend.

It's like we know a secret and we giggle, but I've forgotten what the secret is.

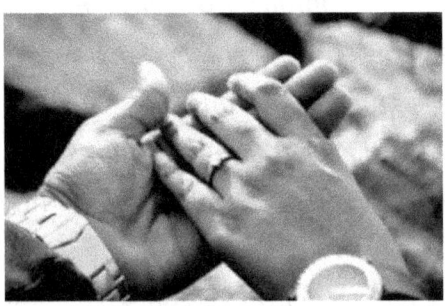

THERE is the hunger for food, and few here seem to have it - they merely eat because it's time and it is expected of them. And the shattered strands of memory cling to ritual as the last bastion of things half remembered.

But there is another hunger - the hunger for love, the hunger to be noticed. It is this hunger that make so many suffer here, though their tongues are incapable of saying what their hearts feel.

Mum feels it as much as any, but she seems more able than most to see it in others.

She can be seen at times coaxing stubborn old

gentlemen to the dinner table - men who have refused to move for staff. You can see the lights return to their eyes, for what gentleman can refuse the proper request of a lady?

And she can be seen holding a hand, or fumbling with a tissue to dry a tear, or urging people indoors, people who have sat in the sun too long.

And there are nights when she cannot be settled herself until she has seen all the other residents (who have become her relatives, school friends, church friends) tucked in and settled for the night.

And so it goes... little forgotten-next-moment acts of kindness for those who hunger for it.

An angel with broken wings is still an angel.

SUMMER has dropped into the courtyard, bringing with it a crispness and a vitality to leaf and flower. The sun floods in, not too hot. Just right. A perfect picture. But someone is there. Mum.

She stands stock still. Clenched fists hang by her side. I look closer. Something has shattered inside her. What tragedy, what suffering could do that to her face?

Tears run down her cheeks and dampen her blouse. She doesn't seem to notice.

A sound. Someone comes. It's Hal. Big, clumsy, genial Hal. Silent Hal. The patient who rarely gets out of his chair, rarely wakes.

Mum used to think he was her father. Now she thinks he is her husband.

Hal has found a chair. He pushes it, scraping, across the concrete patio. He has forgotten how to lift and carry. He pushes it along the ground, bumping it, now, across the grass.

He has remembered her sadness for an extraordinary time and his eyes reflect her suffering. He is bringing her the chair.

"This will fix her," he says. Rare, intelligible words.

It is not so much a chair he is bringing, but something from the heart.

His eyes change. Confusion. So near and yet so far. What was it he was doing? Something. Doesn't matter. He sits on the chair and tries to remember and dozes off.

Peace and tragedy share a courtyard on a beautiful day in summer.

#

HOW can anyone understand what a person with dementia suffers? How can we feel what they feel?

In the last year of mum's life, my own health suffered, and suffered in a way that helped me comprehend mum's plight more fully.

I was already physically disabled, but now mental health suffered. The weight of looking after dad and mum, of coping with my own physical health and with family deception, plus the stress of watching Judy suffer and of having to give up my writing was too much. I suppose you'd say I had a kind of breakdown.

I became very forgetful. I could not concentrate. I could focus on nothing. I could not write. I could not read. I could not do simple mathematics. I was unable to think logically through anything and I became very tired, bone weary, all the time.

I'll say no more than that, because I'm still struggling and I don't want to bring it all back.

Suffice to say that, as part of it, I was diagnosed as having Clinical Depression and went on to medication. The treatment proved, for me, worse than the condition. Eventually I threw the medication away and

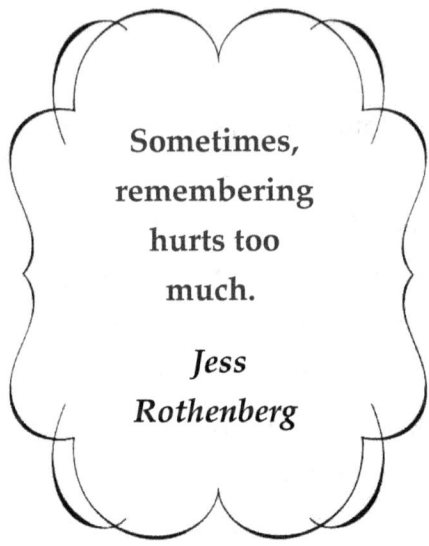

Sometimes, remembering hurts too much.

Jess Rothenberg

I gradually came out of it. But I can't say I've ever totally recovered and I'll never recover that lost year.

I suppose you could say that I went through, and am still going through, to a lesser degree, some small part of what mum was going through.

Today, fear hovers in the back of my mind. Fear that I have sipped the Broth of Oblivion and am destined to lose my future. I try to shake it off, as mum must have tried to shake it off, but the feeling persists, and it is too horrible to contemplate.

I'll change the subject. I'll talk about the family deception.

#

WHY do we do to each other the things we do? Is there not enough heartache in the world without creating our own? Must it be part of the process of coping with stress to lash out at those we love, or should love?

In my case, some members of my family - slap bang in the middle of mum's illness - tried to take dad out of our home, away from Judy and me, away from our care. Why? To this day I have no idea.

But I do know this: the whole affair hurt me as much as anything I can remember in my life.

Dad needed our constant care. He had cancer, he'd had a heart attack and a stroke. He had renal failure and congestive cardiac failure. He'd had a hip replacement and had degenerative spinal disease. He had emphysema. He was almost deaf and had poor eyesight. He fell often. He had leg ulcers. In the later stages, he had savage diarrhoea. He was a sick man.

We knew what to look for, knew his medications, knew how to care for him. In fact, I had told him we would care for him until it became impossible for us, or until the doctors said he could have better care elsewhere.

And the family wanted to take him away and put him in a nursing home, like mum. By deception. By stealth. (You will remember that some of the family actually succeeded in abducting him a year later).

How did we find out about the plot? Judy and I were working in an office at the back of our home. From here we could see dad through the window of his bedroom (when he was in that room). We knew someone was coming to the house, because my sister, who was visiting from Queensland, had been flustered, cleaning dad's area all morning. But we were not told anything. Then my brother arrived. We always tried to give dad his privacy, and we waited for an invitation to join them, but it didn't come.

Then two women arrived. We knew immediately who they were. They were from the Aged Care Assessment Team. They could only be there because they had been invited to assess dad for nursing home placement. You can't get into a nursing home in Australia without this assessment.

They left. My brother left. Without saying hello. We asked what was happening. Dad and my sister said my brother wanted to get dad into the same nursing home mum was in; that he had arranged it. My sister denied knowing anything about it until my brother arrived that day. The lies we tell.

We questioned dad gently. My brother, he said, had said it would be good for him to be with mum. But we knew that dad could not be placed with mum, because he could not gain a place in a secure dementia ward. There was no way he could be assessed as such.

As it turned out, he had been told this by the ACAT members during their visit, but my brother assured dad he could get him a place in the building next to mum's. We checked. Yes, he could, but that building was farther away than dad could walk, and by this time, he was in a wheelchair for anything over about ten paces. We offered to buy him an electric scooter, but he was afraid of operating it. There was no way he could go to that place and see mum. He would have to wait for Judy and I to come and take him. What was the point? Dad decided to stay with us.

For reasons that remain way beyond comprehension, my family tried to take dad away from our care. Did they think we were doing a bad job? They had thought nothing through. I was dad's formal carer, legal guardian and held his power of attorney, so he could go nowhere without my approval. Yet they tried

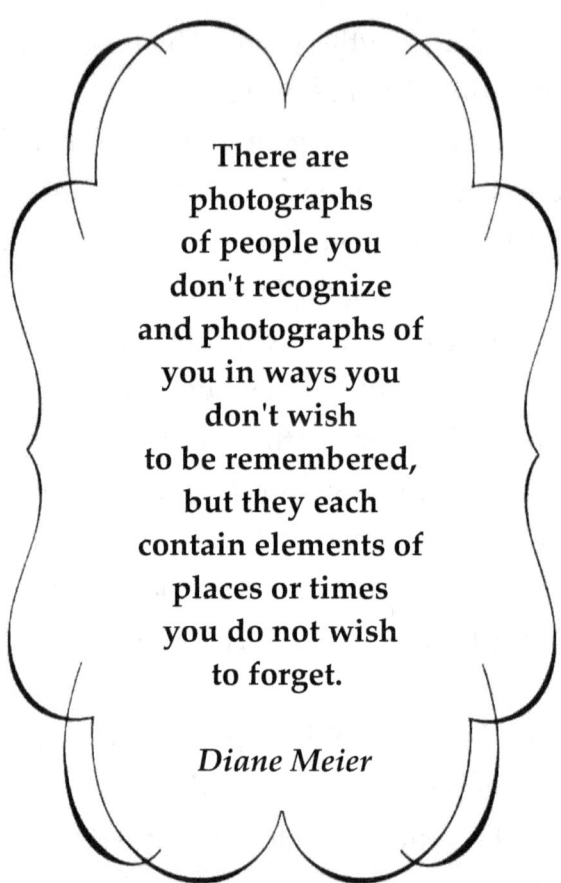

There are
photographs
of people you
don't recognize
and photographs of
you in ways you
don't wish
to be remembered,
but they each
contain elements of
places or times
you do not wish
to forget.

Diane Meier

to move him by stealth.

And, worst of all, they built up the hopes of a sick, old man that he could be with his wife one last time. Nothing hurts quite like betrayal, but forget my anguish over the affair. Think of dad's when he was let down. How could they do such a thing? How could they? The blanket of secrecy has come down, and I will never know.

#

WHAT courage does it take to fight on when you know you cannot win?

It takes courage to fight the screaming enemy on the battlefield, but how much more does it take to fight the silent, invisible, insidious enemy in the mind?

Someone once said the fight is no less noble because there is no drummer marching ahead of you as you face the day's battle, and no crowds at day's end shouting your return from victory or defeat.

Few are brave enough to fight day after day, heartbreak after heartbreak, alone and lonely.

In the world of dementia, no-one can fight your battle for you, no matter how much they want to.

And there can be no doubt that mum's long preparation for death was a much greater torment for her than the eventual suffering of that death.

John F. Kennedy once said that, to find courage, we must each look deep into our own soul.

Who will ever know to what depths mum had to

plunge? All we know is that she found what she was looking for, what she needed. She found courage. Almost incomprehensible courage.

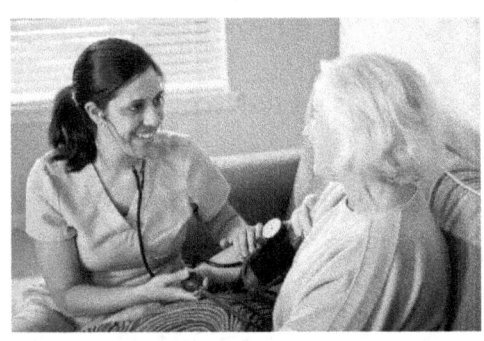

THERE were periods in which she refused to take to her bed. These were the times when she was physically ill, when her failing heart protested at its load. She would struggle for breath and rub her chest, where the angina brought her pain, and she would try to fan away the clammy heat that enveloped her.

She would refuse to lie down. To lie down might mean sleep and from sleep there might be no awakening.

At times like these, when nurses saw the fear, they would keep vigil with her - all night if necessary - comforting her, stroking her, keeping that Grim Reaper at bay.

Eventually, she would drift into a sitting up sleep, knowing that God, and His nurses, were awake.

Until you look into the dark recesses of life, you don't realize how many beautiful souls there are on this planet.

SHE had her own moon phases, waxing and waning between black despair and deeper forgetfulness, which never brought hope, but did bring, on occasion, a kind of contentment.

There were periods of dark fear, almost to the stage of panic, then glimpses of light, when nursing staff could reach her and comfort her.

During these reaching phases, these angels of mercy worked less on her body and more on her spirit, preparing her for what was to come. Preparing her for death.

And, though they did very well for her physically, it was in this quiet, non-religious but spiritual healing that they excelled. This was heart-to-heart stuff, administered with love and received with love. It was God's work. No-one asked them to do it, but it was needed and they responded as only truly beautiful souls can.

I will never forget those nurses at Carrington Nursing Home at Camden.

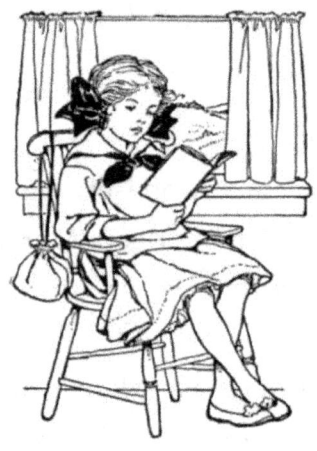

SHE shed garments until she was a picture again of elegance and simplicity. The overcoat of deception slid from her shoulders and she slipped out of the heavy gloves of fault-finding. She put aside the gaudy beads of pretense and the flowery dress of illusion.

She had returned to an age of innocence, to an age where beauty was forever.

Did we love her then because she smiled the innocent smile of a child, or did she smile in innocence because she somehow perceived we loved her?

#

BIRDS sing after a storm. But who will sing if the storm seems without end?

Surely the longest day must have its end. Even the most miserable night inevitably gives way to first light.

Time, the enemy, becomes time, the friend. The inexorable lapse of minutes and hours and weeks and months drags the weary soul towards a new dawn, an eternal sunrise.

If a seed buried in the darkness of the soil can burst forth one day towards the sun and turn into a beautiful flower, what of the soul buried in despair? Can it not, by some miracle of faith, burst forth one day towards God?

This has become my prayer. My constant prayer.

Lord, let the suffering end.

#

AT last she learnt to let go. She knew. Home was suddenly not where she had once lived, or where she wanted to live, but where her soul was going.

It was not the surrender of cowardice that she

succumbed to, finally - it could never be that with mum - but a letting go, an opening up, a release of the spirit.

She had fought the good fight, run the race. It was time to rest. Time to let go.

Time to wait peacefully for God.

WE visited her on that last Sunday and she looked dreadful. She was still in bed, which was most unusual, and we could not rouse her. We called for the nurse, who managed to wake her.

Mum, without having time to even think about it, said: "I think I'll have to go to Mass later."

"Yes, Kathleen," said the nurse, "but you have visitors now."

Mum looked at us blankly. Then, out of some far away mist of instinct or memory, she remembered her manners.

"I must get up," she said, and she insisted on it.

The nurse helped her to rise and brush her hair at the mirror. She was very weak.

"A little more over here," she said, and the nurse obliged.

"That's better," said the one who remained conscious of the niceties until the end.

The mirror showed what life had done to her, but not what she had done in return. The mirror could not show her that life is better for the most insignificant soul having passed through it.

It occurred to me at that moment that nothing on earth - nothing - can wipe out the influence of a pure, simple life devoted to raising a family. The shadow of that influence will fall in places the original soul never trod, in ways it never imagined.

We will never know what debts the world owes to simple souls like mum.

The mirror on that Sunday morning could not show the beautiful thoughts, the great deeds, the thriving love that would come into the world because mum came before. Her seed through the generations would produce unimagined blossoms in life's garden.

But she could only think of her hair. And Judy.

I mentioned that mum always remembered Judy's name more than any other in the family. And she remembered her on this last Sunday of her life.

She motioned Judy to come closer, and whispered in her ear: "Thank you, Judy, for coming to see me and looking after me. And thank you for bringing the boys to see me."

"The boys" were dad and myself. She didn't remember us, but she remembered Judy.

And she remembered her manners.

#

A MAN called William Shakespeare had something to say in *As You Like It* about the various stages of life:

Last scene of all,
That ends this strange eventful history,
Is second childishness and mere oblivion,
Sans teeth, sans eyes, sans taste, sans everything.

Mum had been losing her teeth, and finding them again, for two years; she could not read or see detail because she kept losing her glasses or thought she didn't need them; she had long ago lost the taste for food; she had lost her lifestyle and her life, everything.

What we took of hers from the nursing home was pitiful.

She left little money behind, nothing of heirlooms

or worldly goods or measurable value.

But what she did leave were generations of souls each carrying her traits, her spiritual values, her essence.

In this way, she left the world treasure beyond price.

AND, although the world has long revered Shakespeare as among the wisest of the wise, mum, deep at heart, knew that he was wrong about the "last scene of all".

Mum had been taught from childhood, and always believed, that the last scene of life is not oblivion, but eternity.

And God shall wipe away all tears from [her] eyes; and there shall be no more death, neither sorrow, nor crying, neither shall there be any more pain: for the former things are passed away.
John the Devine.

#

THAT is the essence of what I remember of mum's life when she could no longer remember it.

What follows next is the rest of mum's story as I like to think of it.

The Angel of Memory

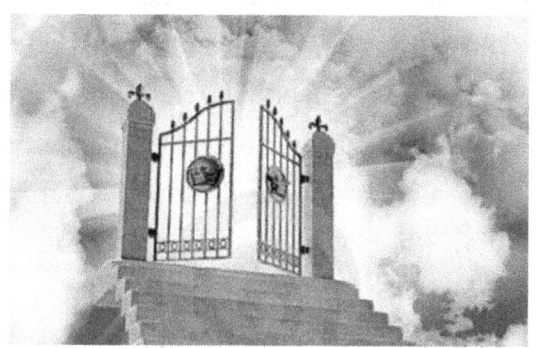

ON All Saints Day, 2002, a new soul arrived at the Pearly Gates seeking admission. She was frail and hesitant, and was overawed when she was greeted by St Peter himself.

The light all around was dazzling and the big man was intimidating with his deep voice, the staff in his hand, and the Golden Keys dangling at his waist. A host of attending angels fluttered about, busy processing the new arrivals.

"Ah, Kathleen Patricia Morgan," Peter said. "We've been expecting you. Yes, indeed."

There was nowhere for Kathleen to hide, and, to be

truthful, although she was shy in such company, her initial awe had vanished, for some reason, and she was no longer really afraid. So she stood and smiled and tried to remember her social graces while Peter studied entries in the Great Book of Records.

"I see here that you were rich," said Peter.

"Oh no," said Kathleen, startled. She remembered something about it being harder for a camel to pass through the eye of a needle than for a rich person to enter heaven. "You must be confusing me with someone else."

Peter glanced at her, amusement playing at his eyes and the corners of his mouth. "No confusion here," he said. "But I'm not talking of money or riches in worldly goods. I'm talking about the much rarer spiritual values. In these, you are wealthy indeed."

Kathleen just looked at him, trying to comprehend.

"You are rich," Peter said, "in kindness, friendship, self-sacrifice, courage, honour and nobility of spirit. And you are especially treasured here because you shared these values with your family."

"Oh," said Kathleen, raising her head and straightening an already straight back.

"I see you were married for 65 years," the gatekeeper said. "According to the record, your happiness began when you married the one you loved, and blossomed when you loved the one you married."

Peter laughed. "These angels really have a way with words," he said.

Kathleen smiled, but, in truth, she was a little dizzy trying to take it all in.

"They are not only a bit fanciful with words," Peter said, "but they also tend to overlook certain things in their reports. I think they have a bit of a selective memory themselves."

He looked at Kathleen and smiled. "However, as they put it, you created a home in which superfluities were not required and necessities were not wanting. Admirable. Admirable."

"Well," said Kathleen, who never liked to play second fiddle in a conversation, "home and family were everything. Home was always more than a roof to keep out the rain and walls to keep out the wind."

Peter held up his hand.

"You have seen three generations started, with countless more to come," he said. He knew better than to let her get going, and he had a long waiting list of applicants to get through. "You created families where home was a place for children to grow up in warmth and safety."

"Yes," said Kathleen, warming to her task and quickly regaining top form. "Home is where children learn what is right, what is good and what is kind. It's where you go for comfort, or when you're sick. It's where joy is shared and sorrow eased. Where children are wanted. Where the simplest food is good enough for kings, because it has been earned. Where..."

"Bless you," said Peter. He was losing control. He had to stop the gathering snowball of her talking. He knew what many on earth did not, that the greatest thing anyone can do for humanity is to bring up a family. A mother's heart, he thought, is a child's playroom, schoolroom, sickroom, chapel and refuge.

"The record tells us you were willing to sacrifice every comfort for your children's benefit, surrender every pleasure to their enjoyment," he said. He knew the record was selective, but, if you couldn't be selective here, where could you be? "You gloried in the slightest hint of their fame and exalted in every glimpse of their prosperity. And, if adversity overtook any of them, your arms were always open."

Now even Kathleen was silent. This was higher

praise than she ever dreamed of giving herself. Perhaps she would get through the gates after all.

"And another thing," said Peter. "You never looked for God in the burning bush, in the parting of the sea, or in the thunderous voice from heaven. Instead, you learnt to look for the miraculous and the hand of God in the day-to-day events of your life."

Peter slammed the book shut and looked at her.

"I've read enough," he said. "In all your forgetting, you never forgot God. Now He has not forgotten you."

"Well, I have been worried sick," said Kathleen. "I have had terrible trouble with my memory. I can't remember things."

"Yes, we know all about that," said Peter, as he waved to an angel hovering nearby.

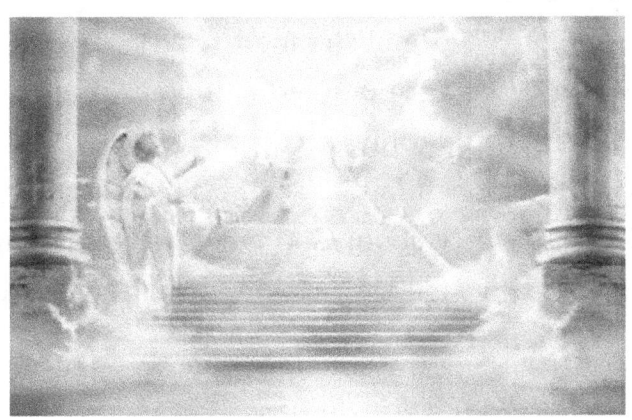

The angel, with apricot-colored wings, brighter and more cheerful than the rest, fluttered over.

"I'm the Angel of Memory," she said. "I'll take care of you. I've been assigned to you for some time."

"Oh," said Kathleen. This was not how she had imagined things when the nuns spoke of angels.

"As a matter of fact," said the angel, "I'm the one who gave you glimpses of memories over the past few years, when you needed cheering up. It's been my job to count your tears and whisper you a song of joy for every one of them."

"Oh," said Kathleen. "That's so kind. So very kind. But, tell me, how can I face God when I can't remember things? What if I've disappointed Him? What if He's not pleased with what I've done, or not done?"

The angel took her hand.

"Haven't you been listening to Peter?" she asked. "How can God be disappointed with your record?"

Kathleen could only shrug. There were surely things not mentioned in the Great Book of Records?

"But let's worry about God when we get to Him," the angel said. She smiled, stroking Kathleen's hand.

"As to memory," she said, "it was never really lost, you know."

"But I *have* lost my memory. Will God give it back?"

"No," said the angel, smiling. "Your memory was never lost. Your loved ones remember everything. They have treasured memories that will never fade."

As the angel spoke, Kathleen realized they had entered the gates of Heaven.

"You are now in heaven," the angel announced, making it sound like the Prize of Prizes it truly was. "From this moment on, you will never forget what you wish to remember, and never remember what you should forget."

Kathleen was radiant and felt a lightness of being she had never experienced. The weight of the world had dropped from her.

"And no," said the angel, "God won't have to give you back your memories. He will leave that to your loved ones. Every time they pray and talk to you, they will remind you of all the beautiful, loving things that have happened throughout your life. As long as any of them live, you will relive another beautiful memory every day."

As they walked, Kathleen began to glow with joy. The angel squeezed her hand.

"Speaking of loved ones..."

Quite suddenly, as if they had appeared out of nowhere, people were all around them and there was a great buzz in the air. Kathleen was taken aback. She looked, and looked again, and her heart leapt.

"Mum, dad..." she said, and that is all she could get out.

They were all there. Bert, with his face of old. Arthur. The sisters. School friends, church friends, neighbors. All the lost ones, found again. They were all there. So many.

The angel took Kathleen's arm and the whole throng moved on, walking towards God.

And God was smiling.

A Final Word

IF YOU liked this book, could I ask you to do something for me to help promote it? I love writing about subjects that I think might leave readers feeling good about themselves and the world they live in. But I need help to let future readers know about my books.

My books cannot be found in bookstores (unless they are ordered in), but can be found online at amazon.com. (Bookshops, libraries and other outlets can stock the books by ordering through the printer, CreateSpace, at www.createspace.com). Since it's not normally in bricks and mortar stores, I have to find ways to let people know about it. If you could help me in this task, you would provide a very helpful service for future readers.

One of the best ways to promote books these days is to go to the Amazon website, search for books by title or author's name, and post a comment or review or just a few words that might help people decide whether to buy it or not. (My website has a direct link to the various books to make it easier.)

Any mention in social networks or book clubs and so on would also be very helpful. I think you know more than I do about spreading the word to friends, and I'm sure you'd be more comfortable talking about my books than I am.

I'd also like to hear from you any thoughts or advice or reviews or comments you may have. You can contact me directly at any time by email at brianmorganbooks@gmail.com.

Thank you for reading and for any support you might feel you are able to give. My website at www.brianmorganbooks.com has other reviews and testimonials, plus details of all of my books. I hope you get the opportunity to enjoy and benefit from my other books as time goes by.

Brian

About the Author

BRIAN MORGAN is an award-winning, best-selling writer, who is dedicating the senior years of his life to inspiring and motivating people through his books and other writings.

He has been described as a business and thought leader, a business founder, an integrity advocate, a national award-winning journalist, editor and publisher, and an internationally acclaimed author.

He has also been honoured by his community on numerous occasions for his long service to various community groups and organisations.

In 2012, in association with The Writers Trust, he started a program to publish all of his books in print and as eBooks. All the details can best be found on his website, www.brianmorganbooks.com.

Brian's new mission in life is summed up in his site's logo: *Stories to Touch Lives.*

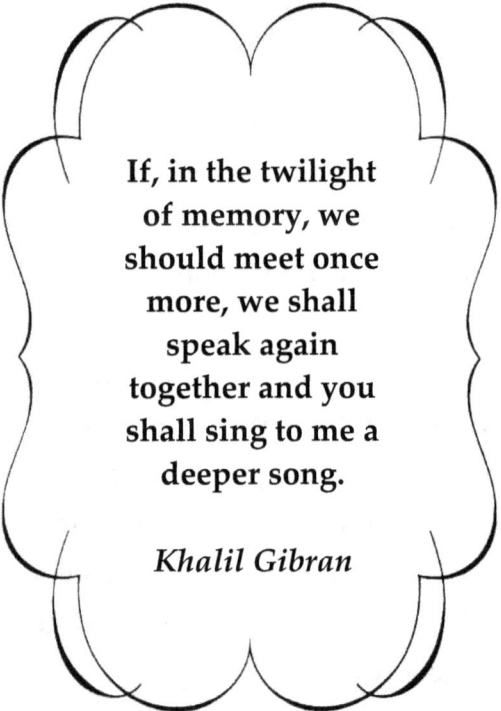

If, in the twilight of memory, we should meet once more, we shall speak again together and you shall sing to me a deeper song.

Khalil Gibran